Acupuncture

PATTERNS & PRACTICE

Li Xuemei & Zhao Jingyi

EASTLAND PRESS ◆ SEATTLE

Copyright © 1993 by Zhao Jingyi and Li Xuemei

Published by Eastland Press, Inc.
P.O. Box 99749
Seattle, WA 98139, USA
www.eastlandpress.com

All rights reserved. No part of this book may be reproduced or transmitted in any form or by any means, electronic or mechanical, including photocopying, recording, or by any information storage and retrieval system, without the prior written permission of the publisher, except where permitted by law.

Library of Congress Catalog Card Number: 92-85309
ISBN-13: 978-0-939616-78-7

2   4   6   8   10   9   7   5   3   1

Book design by Gary Niemeier

Contents

Foreword

ACUPUNCTURE AND MOXIBUSTION are essential aspects of Chinese medicine, which has become one of the most effective medical therapies in the world.

The unique theories of acupuncture were developed in China over a long period and the authors of *Acupuncture Patterns and Practice,* Doctors Li Xuemei and Zhao Jingyi, are worthy inheritors of this great tradition. They graduated from the Beijing College of Chinese Medicine in both Western and Chinese medicine, and over the years have benefited much from the many specialists with whom they have worked and studied.

The book that they have written offers in great detail the unique concepts and diagnostic procedures of Chinese medicine. It is professionally written and displays the authors' wide knowledge of Chinese medicine. I welcome Dr. Li's and Dr. Zhao's contribution to the promotion of Chinese medicine worldwide.

—*Dr. Tian Conghuo*
Chief Researcher, National Academy of Chinese Medicine
Senior Consultant, Guang An Men Hospital, Beijing, China
Assistant Secretary-General, Chinese National Association of
   Acupuncture-Moxibustion

Acknowledgements

WE WOULD LIKE TO THANK and express our appreciation to all our teachers, professors, and friends who have helped us.

We greatly appreciate the training we received at the Beijing College of Chinese Medicine. We would especially like to mention Professors Song Tianbin, Liu Duzhou, Wang Mianzhi, Ren Yingqiu, Lu Zhaolin, and Yang Weiyi.

For clinical training we were lucky to have as our teachers the best specialists in acupuncture and internal medicine. Consultants from the affiliated hospital of the Beijing College of Chinese Medicine, Doctors Jiang Jijun, Zhang Guorui, He Shuhuai, Jiao Shude, Wang Yongyan, and doctors from the China Academy of Chinese Medicine, Li Zhiming, Ye Chenggu and Zhong Meiquan, gave us the benefit of their great knowledge. Under their guidance we gained much practical experience, and they encouraged us to pursue our careers in teaching and practice.

We would like to specially mention Professor Tian Conghuo, Director of the Acupuncture Department of Guang An Men Hospital attached to the China Academy of Chinese Medicine, who gave much of his time to check the manuscript and who has kindly written the foreword to this book.

We are greatly indebted to Dr. Josephine Freeney for all her hard work in connection with the book and with the English. We would also like to thank Michael Cawley for his help with the English, and Charles Gannon for reading and correcting the proofs.

We appreciate the expert advice and excellent editing of Dr. Dan Bensky and John O'Connor of Eastland Press.

Finally, we would like to acknowledge the help and support of our friends, Dr. Primoẑ Roẑman of Slovenia, Vick E. Martin of New Zealand, Helen Mahoney, Helen Murrie, and Christopher Bourke of Australia, and Fred M. Stern and Melanie King of the United States.

Preface

PATTERN PRACTICE is an important part of the study of Chinese medicine as it helps students and practitioners apply basic theory to clinical practice, and improves their ability to diagnose and treat patients.

We feel that a book devoted to clinical pattern practice is needed in addition to the general textbooks in basic theory that are currently available. For the would-be practitioner who is about to embark on clinical practice, this material is essential.

Through actual case studies, this book offers an understanding of how Chinese medical theory and classical philosophy work in the clinic. We have collected the cases that form the basis of this book during several years of practice and teaching. The cases are grouped in chapters under appropriate headings, and for each case we have detailed the history, diagnosis, method of treatment, follow-up, and points of significance for teaching purposes.

This book can be used for teaching, as a means of testing one's self, or as a reference book by students or practitioners of any level. We advise the reader to follow the guidelines set forth here in order to develop a good technique for analyzing one's own cases.

The book is suitable for readers who have a basic knowledge of Chinese medicine and acupuncture. Our aim is to instruct the reader in how to put the basic theories of Chinese medicine into practice. Charts which summarize the method for diagnosing each type of disorder are provided at the end of chapters. These charts will help practitioners improve their diagnostic skills.

We sincerely hope that this book will be helpful for our readers in improving their knowledge in this field.

Common Cold

CASE 1: **Male, age 30**

Main complaint	Fever
History	Two-day history of fever. The patient was exposed to cold in the course of a business trip. He felt cold and had an aversion to cold. His temperature was 38.6°C. There was nasal obstruction with watery nasal discharge, an absence of sweating, no sore throat but a slight cough with some white sputum, and generalized aching. He was not thirsty. His appetite was poor. Urination and bowels were normal.
Tongue	Slightly red body, thin, white, rather moist coating
Pulse	Floating and a little tight
Analysis of symptoms	1. Feeling chilled, accompanied by fever— invasion of superficial tissues by pathogenic factors. 2. Absence of sweating—obstruction of the pores. 3. Nasal obstruction with watery nasal discharge, cough with white sputum— obstruction of Lung qi. 4. Generalized aching—poor movement of qi in the channels. 5. Light red tongue with thin coating and floating pulse—exterior pattern. 6. White, moist coating, tight pulse—cold.
Basic theory of case	In Chinese medicine there are six important environmental factors: wind, cold, summerheat, dampness, dryness, and fire. Under certain conditions these natural factors can become pathogenic, i.e., cause disease. Each pathogenic factor has different characteristics, thus the signs and symptoms caused by each of them are likewise different. Cold is one of the most common pathogenic factors. Among its characteristics are the following: • Cold is a yin pathogenic factor. It obstructs the circulation of yang qi, and also readily consumes the yang of the body. • Cold has a tendency to 'freeze' and therefore to slow down circulation of qi and blood, leading to obstruction in the channels.

• Cold is characterized by constriction, which closes the pores in the skin and constricts the interstices and pores, leading to an absence of sweating. Constriction in the channels and collaterals results in generalized aches and pains, while muscle spasm occurs when there is constriction of the muscles and sinews.

Cause of disease

Pathogenic cold

There is a clear history of exposure to cold, and the symptoms include aversion to cold with an absence of sweating and generalized aching. These symptoms imply that the protective qi and the pores are blocked by the cold, leading to poor circulation of qi and blood in the channels and collaterals.

Site of disease

Superficial tissues, namely the skin, interstices and pores, channels and collaterals.
    The main evidence to support this finding is the aversion to cold and fever occurring together, absence of sweating, light red tongue with thin white coating, and floating pulse.

Pathological change

When external pathogenic factors in the environment invade the body, it is the superficial tissues that are affected first. Under normal conditions the protective qi circulates and spreads over the body surface, regulating body temperature, so that in good health a person does not feel unduly cold.
    In this case the invasion of pathogenic cold has injured the protective qi, interfering with its function and preventing it from reaching the body surface, such that the patient feels cold. The characteristic of this type of cold is that the patient feels cold and may even shiver, but the cold is not alleviated by putting on more clothing.
    There are two reasons why the patient also has a fever. Protective qi is part of the yang of the body and therefore has a tendency to move and to be warm. When it is prevented from reaching the body surface by pathogenic cold, it becomes stagnant and confined to a deeper level of the body, thus producing heat. At the same time, the conflict between the protective (antipathogenic) qi trying to reach the body surface and drive out the pathogenic cold which is blocking its progress also generates heat and raises the temperature. The presence of both fever and aversion to cold is characteristic of the invasion by pathogenic cold.

Fig. 1

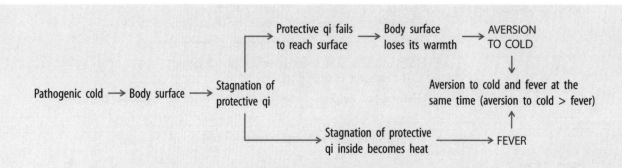

Cold constricts and the patient does not sweat because the pores in the skin are constricted and closed. The tendency of cold to cause constriction or 'freezing' also leads to the stagnation of qi and blood in the channels and collaterals, which in turn causes general aching.
    The Lung governs the skin and body hair and has the function of dispersing the protective qi over the body surface. When there is invasion by pathogenic cold this is no longer possible, so there is a tendency for the Lung qi to stagnate, producing a mild cough. The Lung opens through the nose, thus dysfunction of the Lung in dispersing leads to nasal obstruction and discharge.

A light red tongue with a thin white coating is normal. Here it signifies that the pathogenic factor is only on the surface and has not influenced the function of the Organs. The moist coating likewise indicates that the body fluids are not injured.

The pulse is floating because the pathogenic factor is on the surface of the body, and because cold causes constriction, the pulse is also tight.

Pattern of disease

The pathogenic factor has invaded the superficial tissues but has not affected the Organs, thus this is an exterior pattern.

The patient feels aversion to cold but is not sweating, has white sputum, a white tongue coating, and a tight pulse. These symptoms all indicate cold.

The history is only two days long, and all of the symptoms are caused by invasion of the pathogenic factor, with no obvious injury to the antipathogenic factor or body resistance. The pathogenic factor is strong and this implies a pattern of excess.

Additional notes

1. Why does the patient have a poor appetite?

The Spleen has the function of bringing body fluids and food essence upwards to the Lung. The pathogenic cold has interfered with the Lung's ability to disperse, and this in turn has to some extent affected the function of the Spleen.

2. Is there evidence of an interior pattern in this case?

The Lung's function of dispersing and the Spleen's function of transporting food essence are affected, so why is this an exterior pattern? The pathogenic factor at present is confined to the skin, interstices and pores, channels and collaterals and has not invaded either the Lung or Spleen. The dysfunction of Lung and Spleen are merely secondary to the surface stagnation. They are not the main complaint, and there is no other evidence of an interior problem.

Conclusion

1. According to the eight principles:
   This pattern is exterior, cold, and excessive.

2. According to etiology:
   Invasion of superficial tissues by pathogenic cold.

Treatment principle

1. Expel the pathogenic cold.
2. Relieve the superficial obstruction.

Selection of points

L-7 *(lie que)*
B-12 *(feng men)*
G-20 *(feng chi)*

Explanation of points

L-7 *(lie que)* is the connecting point of the Lung channel which has the function of promoting the dispersing action of the Lung to relieve obstruction in an exterior pattern.

B-12 *(feng men)* is a point on the greater yang channel. Its name means 'gate of wind'. According to the six-stage theory of disease, the greater yang is responsible for the surface of the body. This point regulates the qi in the channel, expels pathogenic wind and cold, and removes obstruction. It is a very good point for treating chills, fever, and aching.

G-20 *(feng chi)*: Here this point is used because it is a meeting point between the lesser yang channel and the yang linking vessel. The yang linking vessel is responsible for yang function and relieves exterior symptoms. It is situated on the nape of the neck and is therefore good for removing headache, obstruction in the channels, and exterior patterns involving stiffness in the upper back and nape.

Combination of points

L-7 *(lie que)* and B-12 *(feng men)*, greater yin and greater yang, responsible for exterior patterns. This combination promotes the dispersing function of the Lung and removes stagnation.

B-12 *(feng men)* and G-20 *(feng chi)*: The names of these two points mean 'gate of wind' and 'pool of wind' respectively. They are strong points for expelling wind-cold from the upper body.

Follow-up

The patient returned two days later when his temperature had become normal. The cough was more pronounced and his appetite was still poor. The other symptoms had disappeared, the tongue coating was white and thicker than before, and the pulse was slightly slippery. This implies that although the pathogenic factors had disappeared, the Lung dysfunction remained, and there was some phlegm. Different points were used:

L-7 *(lie que)*
S-40 *(feng long)*

Two days later the patient was quite well and returned to work.

CASE 2: **Male, age 26**

Main complaint

Sore throat

History

One-day history of sore dry throat with some hoarseness. The patient felt feverish and was sweating slightly with a temperature of 37.8°C. He had some aversion to wind and cold, and there was nasal obstruction but no cough. He also had a headache with dizziness. His appetite and food intake were normal, but he drank more fluid than usual. Sleep, bowels and urination were all normal.

Tongue

Red tip, thin, slightly yellow coating

Pulse

Slightly rapid

Analysis of symptoms

1. Slight aversion to wind and cold with fever—
     invasion of the superficial tissues by pathogenic factors.
2. Mild sweating—inability of the pores to open and close efficiently.
3. Nasal obstruction, sore throat, and hoarseness—
     stagnation and obstruction of Lung qi.
4. Dizziness and headache—pathogenic heat rising to disturb the head.
5. Thirsty with a desire to drink—injury to fluids.
6. Red tongue tip, thin yellow coating, and rapid pulse—heat.

Basic theory of case

Wind-heat, which is present in this case, is one of a group of pathogenic factors which also includes damp-heat, summerheat, and toxic heat. All share the common characteristic of heat. When heat attacks the body it affects the yang aspect first, leading to symptoms in the superficial tissues and the upper part of the body, namely the head, face, throat, and Lung.

Heat also consumes the body fluids, resulting in dehydration, so that symptoms such as thirst, dry throat, and constipation may arise.

Cause of disease

Wind-heat

The patient has a mild aversion to wind and cold with fever and some sweating, which indicates injury to the protective qi and dysfunction of the pores. Symptoms such as headache, sore throat, and nasal obstruction relate to the upper or yang aspect of the body.

Site of disease | Superficial tissues

This is indicated by the aversion to wind and cold, fever, sweating, and the thin tongue coating.

Pathological change | Wind-heat is a yang pathogenic factor which tends to rise and attack the upper part of the body. The Lung is regarded in Chinese medicine as the 'lid' of all the other Organs, and is associated with the exterior, skin, body hair, and pores. It is therefore readily attacked by wind-heat. The Lung opens into the nose via the throat, thus when stagnation of Lung qi is caused by wind-heat, the patient has nasal obstruction and a hoarse voice. When the heat rises and attacks the throat the patient's main complaint is soreness in this area.

The head and face are located on the yang aspect or highest part of the body, which is vulnerable to injury from pathogenic wind-heat. The normal circulation of qi and blood on the head is affected, and the clear yang cannot ascend easily to nourish the face and head. This leads to headache and dizziness.

The patient has a mild aversion to wind and cold, which may give rise to some confusion since the pathogenic factor in this case involves heat. The crucial point is that this is pathogenic heat which is occupying the surface of the body and preventing the natural protective qi from reaching it. The protective qi is stagnated and confined at a deeper level (as in the previous case) and its function of warming and dispersing is thereby impaired. Wind-heat is a yang pathogenic factor that will modify the patient's aversion to cold, but will not play the same role as the body's natural protective qi.

Fig. 2

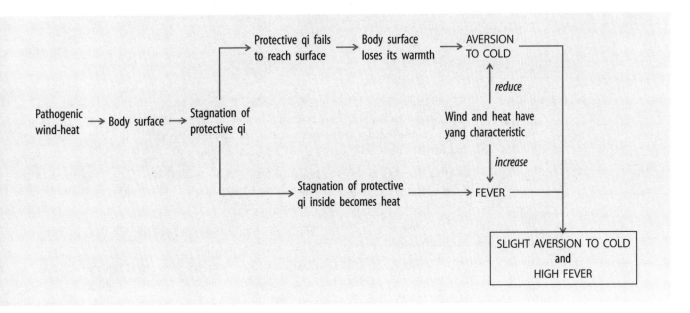

Since wind tends to force open the pores, and heat tends to dilate them, the pores open and sweating occurs. The patient is thirsty and desires to drink because the pathogenic heat has injured the body fluids. The tip of the tongue is red because the heat is in the upper burner; the thin yellow tongue coating indicates that the heat is still superficial. The rapid pulse also reflects the presence of heat.

Pattern of disease | The pathogenic factor remains on the body surface, the tongue body is normal, and its coating is thin. This indicates that the disease has not entered the Organs; it is thus an exterior pattern.

Symptoms such as fever, thirst, red tongue tip with yellow coating, and rapid pulse are all indications of heat.

The history is short and the antipathogenic factor is not injured; it is thus a pattern of excess.

Additional notes

Is there any heat in the Lung?

Because the pattern of heat retained in the Lung shares the symptoms of sore throat, hoarseness, thirst, fever, sweating, and a yellow tongue coating with a rapid pulse, the practitioner may be confused. However, this pattern can be distinguished from wind-heat for several reasons:

- The fever is not accompanied by an aversion to cold, and the patient usually sweats excessively.
- The main symptom is cough with copious yellow sputum, and a stifling sensation in the chest or wheezing.
- The tongue body is red, the tongue coating is not only yellow but also thick and dry, and the pulse is rapid or flooding and rapid.

Retention of heat in the Lung is therefore an interior pattern involving heat and excess, and is thus not present in this case.

Conclusion

1. According to the eight principles:
   This pattern is exterior, heat, and excessive.
2. According to etiology:
   Invasion of the superficial tissues by wind-heat.

Treatment principle

1. Expel the pathogenic wind and heat.
2. Relieve superficial obstruction.

Selection of points

GV-14 *(da zhui)*
LI-11 *(qu chi)*
G-20 *(feng chi)*
SI-17 *(tian rong)*

Explanation of points

GV-14 *(da zhui)* is the meeting point of all the yang channels and is also an important point on the governing vessel. It has a strong function in expelling pathogenic factors from the superficial tissues, especially the yang pathogenic factors. It also relieves obstruction and removes heat in general.

LI-11 *(qu chi)* is the sea point of hand yang brightness. Yang brightness is the channel and Organ which is richest in qi and blood, thus LI-11 *(qu chi)* is appropriate for removing heat and fire.

G-20 *(feng chi)* is used to expel wind, and to relieve symptoms such as headache and dizziness.

SI-17 *(tian rong)* is a local point which removes heat from the throat, resolves swelling, and relieves obstruction and hoarseness. Because it belongs to the hand greater yang channel, it is effective in relieving symptoms associated with exterior patterns.

Combination of points

GV-14 *(da zhui)* and LI-11 *(qu chi)* remove heat. Because GV-14 *(da zhui)* is the meeting of the yang channels and LI-11 *(qu chi)* is a point on the yang brightness channel, they are a strong pair for removing heat and obstruction.

LI-11 *(qu chi)* and G-20 *(feng chi)* are very good points for relieving the headache caused by heat or wind-heat.

Follow-up

The morning following treatment the temperature was normal and the throat only slightly uncomfortable. The following points were then used:

SI-17 *(tian rong)*
G-20 *(feng chi)*

The patient was advised to rest for one more day, after which he completely recovered.

CASE 3: **Female, age 32**

Main complaint	Headache and fever

History   One week ago the weather became colder and the patient neglected to dress warmly. She developed a fever of 38°C with intermittent sweating. When she sweated the temperature went down, but when the sweating ceased the temperature rose. She had an aversion to cold, nasal obstruction with watery discharge, and a headache with a heavy sensation around the head. Her limbs felt heavy and sore. She was not thirsty. Her appetite was poor and she felt nauseated and vomited once after experiencing fullness in the epigastrium. Her stools were unformed, bowel movement once or twice per day, and urination was normal.

Tongue   Pale body with a white, greasy coating, slightly yellow on the root

Pulse   Soft

Analysis of symptoms

1. Aversion to cold and fever—
     invasion of the superficial tissues by pathogenic factors.
2. Intermittent sweating—dysfunction of the pores.
3. Nasal obstruction with watery discharge—stagnation of the Lung qi.
4. Heavy sensation in the head and limbs—
     retention of dampness in the superficial tissues.
5. Fullness in the epigastrium, nausea and vomiting, poor appetite, and unformed
     stool—poor circulation of qi due to retention of dampness in the middle
     burner.
6. Pale tongue with white coating—cold.
7. Greasy tongue coating, soft pulse—dampness.

Basic theory of case   Dampness as a cause of disease can be external or internal, depending on the way in which it attacks the body. Its nature may be either damp-cold or damp-heat. Dampness alone has the following characteristics:

- It is a yin pathogenic factor which readily consumes the yang qi of the body.
- It is a substantial pathogenic factor, heavy and viscous, and may impede the normal circulation of qi, causing stagnation and sometimes even reversal of qi. Dampness also causes a sensation of heaviness when it is retained in different parts of the body.
- Dampness is thick and greasy and is therefore more difficult to remove than the other pathogenic factors; the history is therefore often rather long.
- The Spleen has the function of transporting and transforming water; both external and internal dampness readily injure Spleen qi.

Cause of disease   Pathogenic cold and dampness

The patient has a history of exposure to pathogenic factors, which after one week of intermittent sweating are still present in the body. This fact, accompanied by the symptoms of heaviness in the head and limbs and the digestive problems, suggests that cold and dampness are present.

Site of disease

1. Superficial tissues.
2. Spleen and Stomach.

The aversion to cold with fever and intermittent sweating indicates that the site of disease is on the skin, pores, channels and collaterals.

The poor appetite, fullness in the epigastrium, nausea, vomiting, and loose stools show that the Spleen and Stomach are involved.

Pathological change

Cold and dampness have invaded the surface of the body, confining the protective qi to a deeper layer. As it struggles to reach the surface, heat is produced. Aversion to cold and fever therefore occur at the same time, but since the yin pathogenic factor predominates, the aversion to cold is more marked than the fever.

Sweating means that the yang qi expresses body fluid through the pores. When pathogenic factors invade the body surface, sweating can remove them through the pores, which is one way to expel exterior disease patterns. In order for sweating to be adequate for this purpose, the yang qi must be strong, and there must be sufficient body fluids. If the temperature returns to normal after sweating, this means that the pathogenic factors have been completely expelled and recovery will follow.

Some pathogenic factors are more difficult to remove than others. Dampness has the characteristic of being thick and greasy, and is therefore difficult to remove once it is retained on the body surface. It tends to block the circulation of qi, leading to obstruction in the channels and collaterals. This in turn prevents sufficient yang qi from reaching the body surface to cause enough sweating. The clinical manifestation is that although some sweating occurs, the symptoms associated with pathogenic dampness nonetheless persist. In this case, which is typical, the patient has some sweating but continues to have a high temperature.

Fig. 3

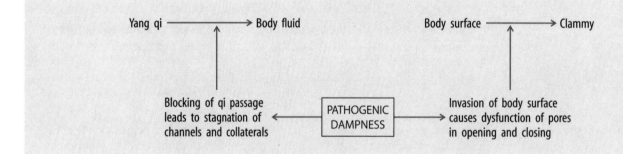

The patient also has a sensation of soreness and heaviness about the face, head, and limbs because the pathogenic dampness retained on the surface of the body impedes the circulation of qi and blood in the channels and collaterals. Thus the clear yang cannot ascend to the head or reach to the body surface in general.

There is nasal obstruction and discharge because the stagnation of protective qi leads to stagnation of Lung qi.

The Spleen is one of the Organs responsible for water metabolism. Pathogenic dampness can interfere with the Spleen qi and cause stagnation of qi in the middle burner, manifested as fullness in the epigastrium. The Spleen's function of digesting food is impaired, leading to poor appetite. The Stomach qi fails to descend and reversal of the flow of qi causes nausea and vomiting. Because the dampness is not properly transported by the Spleen, it goes down to the Large Intestine where it causes loose stools.

The pale tongue and white coating reflect the presence of cold. The greasy quality of the coating and the soft pulse are associated with dampness.

Pattern of disease

Because the pathogenic damp-cold is retained on the body surface the patient has fever and an aversion to cold, indicating an exterior pattern. The dampness has influenced the Spleen and Stomach, meaning that the pattern in this case is also interior.

The patient has an obvious aversion to cold, nasal obstruction with watery nasal discharge, absence of thirst, and a pale tongue with a white coating. The pulse is soft but not rapid. These symptoms reflect a pattern of cold.

The history is not very long, and all the symptoms involve the body surface and the Spleen and Stomach, and are caused by pathogenic dampness. This is a pattern of excess.

Additional notes

1. Is there any evidence of heat in this case?

A white tongue coating indicates cold, while yellow indicates heat. In this case the coating on the root of the tongue is slightly yellow, suggesting that the dampness has a tendency to transform into heat. The dampness blocks the circulation of qi and the yang qi struggles against the dampness, producing heat and causing part of the tongue coating to change from white to yellow. This kind of heat is not strong and is limited to a certain area, thus the general condition of the body is not affected. It can therefore be ignored in terms of diagnosis.

2. Is there Spleen qi deficiency in this case?

The patient has a poor appetite, loose stools, and a pale tongue with a white coating, but the history is short, only one week. These symptoms are caused by dampness obstructing the Spleen and Stomach qi. In the case of Spleen qi deficiency, the history would be much longer and the symptoms more severe.

3. How is invasion by pathogenic cold and dampness distinguished from invasion by cold?

Pathogenic damp-cold and cold are both yin pathogenic factors, and both readily injure the yang qi of the body. When pathogenic damp-cold invades the surface of the body but does not affect the Spleen and Stomach, the primary manifestations will be a severe aversion to cold, a mild fever, and an absence of sweating. The same is true of pathogenic cold.

However, they may be distinguished by the fact that cold causes constriction and hence stagnation and poor circulation of qi and blood in the channels and collaterals, leading to aching in the head and body. Damp-cold, on the other hand, is heavy and greasy, and when it invades the channels and collaterals and interstices and pores, the patient will have very pronounced symptoms of heaviness in the head, trunk, or limbs. Pain is either absent or of little significance.

Conclusion

1. According to the eight principles:
   This pattern is both exterior and interior, but mainly exterior, cold, and excessive.
2. According to etiology:
   Invasion of the superficial tissues by pathogenic cold and dampness.
3. According to Organ theory:
   Impairment of the Spleen and Stomach qi by pathogenic dampness.

Treatment principle

1. Expel the pathogenic cold and dampness and remove the symptoms of the exterior pattern.
2. Remove the dampness and harmonize the middle burner.

Selection of points

GV-14 *(da zhui)*
TB-5 *(wai guan)*
G-20 *(feng chi)*
GV-9 *(zhi yang)*

Explanation of points

GV-14 *(da zhui)* is the meeting point of the seven yang channels and will regulate the qi around the yang channels and strengthen the protective qi in order to expel the pathogenic factors. It can, of course, be used to remove pathogenic heat, but because it acts on the natural resistance of the body, it is also a very good point for expelling other pathogenic factors.

TB-5 *(wai guan)* is the meeting point of the Triple Burner and the yang linking vessels, one of the eight confluent points. Using this point thus causes the qi to flow from the Triple Burner, which is internal, to the yang linking vessel, which is distributed on the yang or external aspect of the body. This improves the circulation of yang qi on the body surface, and tends to push the damp-cold out through the pores. One function of the Triple Burner channel is the regulation of water metabolism; use of this point will thus also remove internal dampness.

G-20 *(feng chi)* is used in this case as a local point because the patient has a heavy sensation around the head with headache. Its use will help remove obstruction and regulate the qi of the head.

GV-9 *(zhi yang)*, a point on the governing vessel, is chosen to remove obstruction from the channels and collaterals by promoting the circulation of yang qi. This point is useful for removing dampness and also in harmonizing the Spleen and Stomach because it is, in effect, a local point. It is an excellent choice in this case because there is both heaviness in the limbs and abdominal symptoms.

Follow-up

This patient was treated daily for three days with the same points. The temperature gradually subsided to normal, but the appetite remained very poor. After three days the points were changed in order to better remove the dampness and harmonize the Spleen:

CV-11 *(jian li)*
S-36 *(zu san li)*
Sp-9 *(yin ling quan)*

These points were used on alternate days for three more treatments, after which the patient felt well.

CASE 4: **Female, age 43**

Main complaint

Bad cold

History

One month ago the patient had a bad cold and has not recovered. She has a feeling of being always cold, with an aversion to wind, and spontaneous sweating. She has a cough with a little sputum but no sore throat or fever. She has general lassitude and fatigue and cold extremities. She is not thirsty. Food intake, bowels, and urine are normal.

The patient has a weak general constitution, easily catches cold, always feels cold, and prefers to wear more clothes than other people.

Tongue

Pale body, white moist coating

Pulse

Sunken, thin, and forceless

Analysis of symptoms

1. Aversion to wind—invasion of the superficial tissues by pathogenic factors.

2. Spontaneous sweating—dysfunction of the pores.

3. Cough with sputum—stagnation of Lung qi.

4. Fatigue, general lassitude, a feeling of being cold, and cold extremities— yang deficiency.

5. Pale tongue with white coating—cold.

6. Sunken, thin, forceless pulse—yang deficiency.

Basic theory of case

Invasion of the body by any external pathogenic factor tends to run a similar course. The onset is acute and the patient recovers naturally within one or two weeks. The history is short and the nature of the disease is excessive.

In the case of a patient with a weak constitution, the antipathogenic factors are not strong enough to expel the pathogenic factors, so they are retained on the body surface. The disease is therefore prolonged.

This type of problem is both deficient and excessive, and represents an important concept in Chinese medicine known as externally-contracted disease with a deficient antipathogenic factor. This means invasion by pathogenic factors with a pre-existing condition of deficiency.

Cause of disease

Pathogenic wind

The patient has a history of easily catching cold, and presently has an aversion to wind with spontaneous sweating, implying that the protective qi has been injured by the pathogenic wind. This patient has no fever, which will be explained later in this discussion.

Site of disease

1. Superficial tissues.
2. Yang qi.

The aversion to wind and the spontaneous sweating indicate that the pathogenic factors have invaded the superficial tissues.

The feeling of being always cold, with cold extremities, fatigue, and general lassitude are evidence of a disorder of the yang qi.

Pathological change

There are two aspects of pathological change in this case: the underlying internal problem and the invasion by external pathogenic factors.

The yang qi of the body includes primary qi *(yuán* or source qi), pectoral qi *(zōng qi)*, nutrient qi *(yíng qi)*, protective qi *(wēi qi)*, the qi of the Organs, and the qi in the channels and collaterals. Protective qi is part of the yang qi of the body, which has the function of warming and nourishing the surface of the body, controlling the opening and closing of the pores, and preventing invasion by pathogenic factors.

Deficiency of protective qi weakens the resistance of the body to disease, such that pathogenic factors frequently enter it, the patient readily catches cold, and recovery is slow. The ability of the yang qi to warm the body is reduced, thus the patient constantly feels cold and wears more clothes than would a healthy person. After invasion by pathogenic factors the yang qi is further consumed, causing the patient to have cold extremities. When there is a deficiency of yang the patient will lack energy and suffer from fatigue and general lassitude. The patient will not be thirsty and may drink less than usual because yang deficiency leads to a pattern of cold in which the body fluids are not consumed.

In this case the main external pathogenic factor is wind. Although wind and cold frequently invade the body together, they in fact have different characteristics. Wind is yang and has a tendency to expand, causing the interstices and pores to open and the body fluids to flow out passively. The main symptoms are therefore an aversion to wind and spontaneous sweating. Cold on the other hand is yin, tends to consume yang, and constricts the interstices and pores. Associated symptoms are an aversion to cold with an absence of sweating, as discussed in the first case of this group.

Here there is an aversion to wind and spontaneous sweating, so the wind has invaded the surface of the body. The presence of this pathogenic factor in the superficial tissues causes stagnation of protective qi, which in turn impairs the dispersing function of the Lung qi. The patient therefore has a cough with sputum. That she has no sore throat indicates that there is no heat present.

The pale tongue with moist white coating indicates the presence of cold. The thin, forceless pulse shows a deficiency of yang, as there is not enough qi to move the blood. The pulse is sunken because of the yang deficiency, and the antipathogenic factor is too weak to rise to the body surface and fight with the external pathogenic factors.

Generally speaking, a patient with an exterior pattern of disease will have an aversion to either cold or wind, accompanied by fever. The fever occurs because the stagnant protective qi transforms into heat. In this case the patient suffers from internal cold caused by deficiency of yang qi. Thus, after the invasion by pathogenic factors, although there is stagnation of qi, it is not strong enough to transform into heat and consequently there is no fever.

Fig. 4

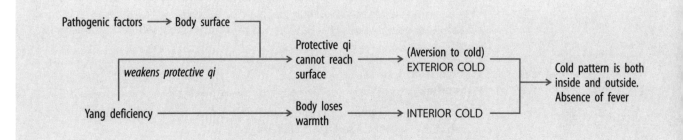

Pattern of disease

The patient has an aversion to wind and spontaneous sweating caused by invasion of pathogenic factors. She also has yang deficiency, with a feeling of being cold and cold extremities. There is thus both an exterior and an interior pattern.

There is no fever, but she has a pale tongue with white coating, and complains of cold extremities: a cold pattern.

There is also yang deficiency with a feeling of being cold, general lassitude, and a thin, forceless pulse, indicating a pattern of deficiency.

Additional notes

1. Usually when there is invasion by external pathogenic factors the onset is acute, the history is short, the pathogenic factors are expelled, and the patient recovers. If this does not occur the pathogenic factors penetrate more deeply and transform into interior heat, with a corresponding worsening in the patient's condition.

In this particular case the patient has yang deficiency, thus the body resistance is too weak to expel the pathogenic factors. At the same time, however, because there is internal cold, there is no reason for the symptoms to transform into a pattern of heat. There is thus a stalemate in which the pathogenic factors are retained on the body surface and the yang deficiency fails to improve.

2. Is this a case of qi deficiency or yang deficiency?

Both qi and yang deficiency can lead to deficiency of protective qi, a condition in which the patient can easily catch cold. This patient has spontaneous sweating, general lassitude, and fatigue, symptoms which are typical of qi deficiency, but she also complains of cold extremities and constantly feeling cold. The correct diagnosis is therefore yang deficiency.

Conclusion

1. According to the eight principles:
   Exterior and interior, cold and deficient.

2. According to etiology:
   Invasion of superficial tissues by pathogenic wind.

3. According to yin-yang theory:
   Yang deficiency.

Treatment principle	1. Expel the pathogenic wind, remove the exterior pattern. 2. Tonify the yang and resolve the interior cold.
Selection of points	CV-6 *(qi hai)* with moxa box S-36 *(zu san li)* with warm needle TB-5 *(wai guan)* B-12 *(feng men)*
Explanation of points	CV-6 *(qi hai)* is effective for tonifying the yang qi and strengthening the Kidney. It also regulates the qi of the entire body.

Explanation of points

CV-6 *(qi hai)* is effective for tonifying the yang qi and strengthening the Kidney. It also regulates the qi of the entire body.

S-36 *(zu san li)* tonifies the yang qi of the entire body, and strengthens and harmonizes the middle burner.

B-12 *(feng men)* expels pathogenic wind and cold and relieves exterior conditions. It also regulates the qi around the greater yang channel.

TB-5 *(wai guan)* is a meeting point of the Triple Burner with the yang linking vessel, and is used to improve the circulation of yang qi on the body surface to aid in expulsion of pathogenic factors.

Combination of points

CV-6 *(qi hai)* and S-36 *(zu san li)* are both very important tonifying points. CV-6 *(qi hai)* is closely related to the Kidney and S-36 *(zu san li)* to the middle burner, both of which are important sources of qi. When moxa is used this pair of points tonifies the yang of the body.

TB-5 *(wai guan)* and B-12 *(feng men)*: TB-5 *(wai guan)* assists the yang qi in reaching the body surface, and B-12 *(feng men)* is effective in removing the wind and cold.

Techniques

With regard to the moxibustion used in this case, the warm needle technique was accomplished by using three pieces of moxa stick on S-36 *(zu san li)*. The moxa box was applied for 15 minutes on CV-6 *(qi hai)*.

Follow-up

After three treatments the aversion to wind and spontaneous sweating had been resolved. Because the pathogenic factors were no longer present, the treatment regimen was changed in order to tonify the antipathogenic factor and promote the body resistance. The following points were used:

L-9 *(tai yuan)*
S-36 *(zu san li)* with warm needle
CV-6 *(qi hai)* with moxa box

The patient was treated twice a week for a month after which she had recovered completely. She continued to use a moxa stick at S-36 *(zu san li)* for ten minutes each day on both sides for two more months. She was instructed to hold the stick 4-5cm above the skin, and to move the stick horizontally with small circular motions.

Diagnostic principles for exterior patterns

1. Concept and principal symptoms

In Chinese medicine an exterior pattern is a group of symptoms caused by the invasion of the skin, interstices and pores, channels and collaterals by external pathogenic factors. Characteristic symptoms include concurrent fever and aversion to cold, nasal obstruction and discharge, headache or aching around the body, cough, and sore throat. The tongue coating is thin and the pulse is floating.

The crucial factors in diagnosis are the simultaneous occurrence of fever and aversion to cold, the thin tongue coating, and the floating pulse.

2. General pathological change

The basic pathological change is that the pathogenic factors remain on the body surface and confine the protective qi to a deeper level in the body. The physiological function of protective qi, which pertains to yang, is to warm the body surface, and when the pathogenic factors prevent it from reaching this area, the superficial tissues are not warmed and the patient develops an aversion to cold. In such cases the protective qi has not been weakened, but merely trapped, and it therefore struggles to reach the surface. This struggle produces heat, which manifests in fever.

The pathogenic factors on the surface block the channels, particularly the collaterals, and also affect the Lung qi, resulting in general aching, nasal obstruction, sore throat, and cough. The tongue coating remains thin, and the pulse floating, because the pathogenic factors are only on the surface and have not affected the function of the Organs.

Fig. 5

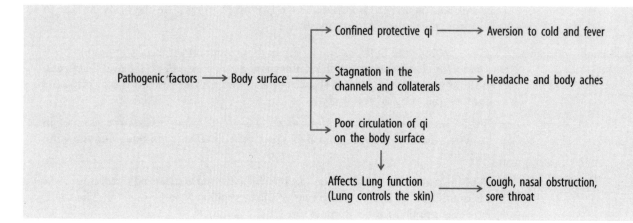

3. Additional points for discussion

i. What is the difference between aversion to cold and feeling cold?

A patient with an aversion to cold has a subjective feeling of cold and may shiver, but the symptoms are not relieved by putting on more clothing. It is always accompanied by fever. This is typical of an exterior pattern.

Some individuals always have a feeling of being cold; they neither shiver nor have a fever, but tend to wear more clothes than most people consider appropriate. The extra clothing relieves their feeling of cold. This is a symptom of yang deficiency, which is an interior pattern. The yang qi has the function of warming the body, thus when it is deficient the patient naturally feels cold. The extra clothing cuts down heat loss from the body surface, and the symptom of feeling cold thus improves. There is, of course, no fever because if anything, the body temperature tends to be below normal.

Fig. 6

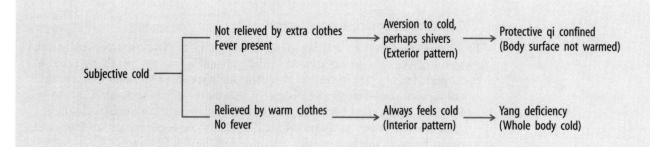

When a patient says that he or she feels cold, it is thus very important to elicit by questioning the precise nature of their symptoms. *See Fig. 6.*

ii. How does one distinguish between different external pathogenic factors?

Invasion of the body by pathogenic factors is the cause of exterior patterns, and in the clinical situation the symptoms must be analyzed in order to determine which factors are present. There are four common patterns: wind-cold, wind-heat, dampness, and dryness.

Fig. 7

WIND-COLD: Marked aversion to cold	Slight or high fever	No sweating, headache, general aching	No thirst	Clear nasal discharge	Cough, white phlegm	No sore throat	Thin, white tongue coating	Floating, tight pulse
WIND-HEAT: Slight aversion to cold	Fever	Little sweating, headache	Slightly thirsty	Yellow nasal discharge	Cough, yellow phlegm	Sore throat	Thin, yellow tongue coating	Floating, rapid pulse
DAMPNESS: Aversion to cold (Symptoms tend to persist)	Fever	Clammy heaviness in head and body	No thirst	Poor appetite, suffocating sensation in epigastric region, nausea or vomiting, diarrhea			Thick, sticky tongue coating	Soft pulse
DRYNESS: Very slight aversion to cold (Dry environment)	Very slight fever	No sweating, seldom pain or aching	Thirsty	Dry nose	Dry cough or very little phlegm	Dry throat	Thin, dry tongue coating	Floating or thin pulse

Additional notes to Fig. 7:

1. There is no sweating in the pattern of wind-cold because cold constricts the pores and prevents the body fluids from passing through.

2. There is thirst in the pattern of wind-heat because pathogenic heat consumes the body fluids.

3. The Spleen is averse to dampness and prefers dryness, thus in the pattern of dampness the Spleen is affected, giving rise to symptoms in the digestive system.

4. In the pattern of dryness, the body fluids are consumed and so there is no sweating, and the patient feels thirsty. The reduction in body fluids also affects the blood, resulting in a thin pulse.

iii. An important concept in Chinese medicine that is relevant here is *xū zhèng wài gǎn bìng,* or 'an externally-contracted disease with a deficient antipathogenic factor.' In the clinical situation it is necessary to ascertain whether the pattern is purely exterior, or whether the patient's antipathogenic factor is also weaker than normal. Purely exterior patterns are excessive, but when a patient previously had a deficiency of antipathogenic factor the pattern will be a mixture of excess and deficiency. There are four types of deficiency, shown below, which give rise to this condition. *See Fig. 8.*

iv. In the clinical situation, how does one decide whether the patient has an exterior pattern?

This is important because if an exterior pattern is present, the first treatment

Fig. 8

principle in Chinese medicine is to remove the pathogenic factors. The entire diagnostic procedure for exterior patterns is shown in Fig. 9.

EXTERIOR PATTERN with QI DEFICIENCY	Susceptible to invasion by pathogenic factors (mainly wind-cold)	Marked aversion to cold, slight or high fever	Spontaneous sweating and wind-cold symptoms	Shortness of breath, general lassitude, forceless pulse, other qi deficiency symptoms
EXTERNAL PATTERN with YANG DEFICIENCY	Susceptible to invasion by pathogenic factors (mainly wind-cold)	Marked aversion to cold, slight or no fever	No sweating and wind-cold symptoms	Fatigue, cold limbs, pale and flabby tongue with white and moist tongue coating, deep and slow pulse, other yang deficiency symptoms
EXTERNAL PATTERN with BLOOD DEFICIENCY	Mainly pathogenic wind-cold or wind-heat invasion	Marked or slight aversion to cold, marked or slight fever	No sweating or sweating, wind-cold or wind-heat symptoms	Pale face and lips, palpitations, pale tongue, thready pulse, other blood deficiency symptoms
EXTERNAL PATTERN with YIN DEFICIENCY	Internal heat and mainly pathogenic wind-heat invasion	Slight aversion to cold and marked fever	Sweating and wind-heat symptoms	Anxiety and feverish sensation in the palms and soles, malar flush, dry stool, red tongue, thready and rapid pulse, other yin deficiency symptoms

Additional notes to Fig. 8:

1. A patient with qi or yang deficiency has lowered body resistance and is therefore easily attacked by wind-cold.
   A patient with yin deficiency and symptoms of heat from deficiency is more prone to invasion by wind-heat, and if they are attacked by other pathogenic factors, the pattern easily transforms into one of heat.

2. A patient with qi deficiency often has spontaneous sweating because the protective qi is weak and cannot control the opening and closing of the pores, thus the body fluid flows out.
   On the other hand, a patient with yang deficiency does not sweat because the cold constricts and closes the pores.
   A patient with yin deficiency sweats because there is an imbalance between the yin and yang of the body, and the heat pushes the body fluids out through the pores.

Fig. 9

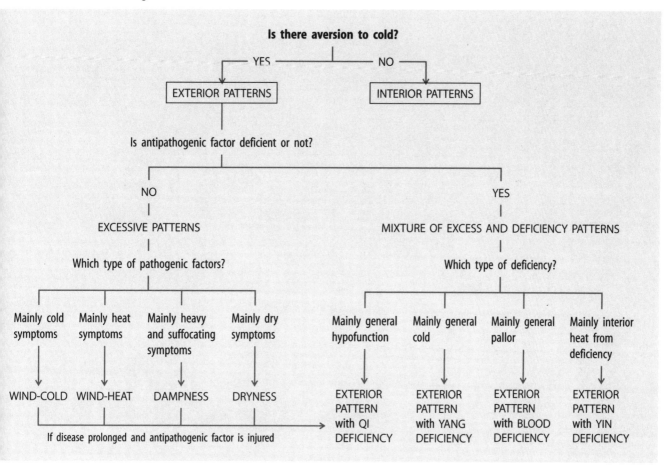

Cough

CASE 5: **Female, age 19**

Main complaint

Cough

History

Two month history of cough, but the symptoms became much worse over the last four days. Originally the symptoms were sore throat and slight cough with white sputum, but four days ago the symptoms changed to severe cough with profuse yellow sputum and chest pain on the right side. The chest pain became worse when she coughed or breathed deeply, and she was admitted to the hospital.

When the patient was admitted she had a temperature of 39.5ºC. She had no aversion to cold and had a feverish sensation around her entire body. The patient had completely lost her appetite, and developed abdominal distention with dryness in the mouth which she relieved by drinking cold water. She felt mentally restless. She had not had a bowel movement for four days, and had yellow urine. Her complexion was red.

Tongue

Red body, yellow and dry coating

Pulse

Slippery and rapid

Analysis of symptoms

1. Cough with yellow, profuse sputum—retention of phlegm-heat.
2. Chest pain—obstruction of qi.
3. Fever, restlessness, yellow urine, and dry stools—heat.
4. Poor appetite and abdominal distention—
   impairment of Spleen's transportive and transformative functions.
5. Red complexion, red tongue, yellow and dry tongue coating—heat.
6. Rapid and slippery pulse—phlegm-heat.

Basic theory of case

The Lung qi has the functions of dispersing and descending. The dispersing function involves moving the protective qi throughout the surface of the body. The Lung also sends qi downward to the Kidney and is thus involved with the metabolism of water in the body. Under normal conditions these two functions of the Lung are cooperative.

Cough is a sign of imbalance within the Lung in dispersing and descending. In Chinese medicine this dysfunction is known as reversal of the Lung qi. There are many possible reasons for this including invasion of external pathogenic factors and internal disorders. Any one or more of the six external pathogenic factors can cause reversal of Lung qi, and there are many substantial pathogenic factors such as phlegm, dampness, and congested fluids which can also be the causative factor. In the clinic the cause must be determined by proper analysis of the symptoms.

Cause of disease

Phlegm-heat

The patient's main symptoms are cough, profuse yellow sputum, thirst, yellow urine, and dry stools, all of which indicate retention of phlegm-heat.

Site of disease

Lung

The patient has a history of cough with excessive phlegm of more than two months' duration. The cough is accompanied by chest pain which intensifies every time she takes a deep breath. All of these symptoms confirm that the site of disease is the Lung.

Pathological change

When external pathogenic factors attack the pores, skin, and interstices the result will be an exterior pattern of disease. If the pathogenic factors attack the Organs, qi, and blood directly, an interior pattern will develop. Or, if the external pathogenic factors on the surface of the body are not resolved, they may progress inward to attack the Organs, qi, and blood, i.e., an exterior pattern may evolve into an interior pattern.

The early stage of disease in this patient showed only symptoms of an exterior nature, e.g., the slight cough and sore throat. During the last two months the patient continued to cough, indicating that the pathogenic factors were retained. The pathogenic factors have now penetrated to the Organ level where they are influencing the Lung's function of dispersing and descending. The cough represents a reversal of the Lung qi. The Lung's function in water metabolism is also interrupted: the congested fluids are retained in the Lungs instead of being sent downwards, leading to retention of phlegm in the Lungs. After a certain period— here two months—the phlegm evolved into a pattern of heat. The phlegm united with the heat to produce a new set of pathogenic factors called phlegm-heat.

This represents a new pattern of disease. One of the primary characteristics of heat is its tendency to rise up, which explains why the cough has become worse and is now accompanied by excessive yellow sputum.

The phlegm blocks the passage of Lung qi and impairs the circulation of qi and blood in the chest, leading to chest pain.

The patient has a fever without any aversion to cold. This is because the source of the heat is internal (Lung) rather than external; thus the heat moves outward to leave the body, causing fever with no aversion to cold.

The Heart and Lung are both located in the chest. The Heart is affected by the heat in the Lung, which accounts for the patient's feverish and restless state. The heat has consumed the body fluids, thus the patient is thirsty with a dry mouth, prefers cold drinks, and has yellow urine with dry stools.

The heat accelerates the circulation of blood and rises to the head where it causes a red complexion and red tongue. The tongue has a dry, yellow coating, which indicates the presence of heat and consumption of the body fluids. The pulse is rapid, indicating heat, and slippery, indicating retention of the pathogenic factors. *See Fig. 1.*

Pattern of disease

Interior

The main indicators of this pattern are retention of phlegm-heat in the Lung, severe cough, and a high temperature with no aversion to cold.

The primary symptoms of heat are yellow sputum, restlessness, thirst, preference for cold drinks, yellow urine, dry stools, red complexion, red tongue, yellow tongue coating, and rapid pulse.

Fig. 1

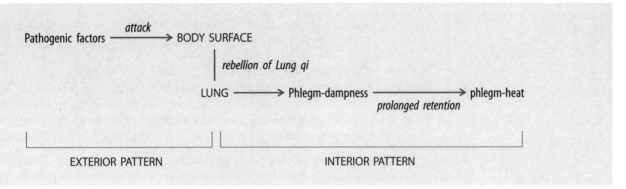

All of the symptoms are caused by retention of pathogenic factors in the Lung. It is thus an excessive pattern of disease.

Additional notes

1. Is there any evidence that an exterior pattern remains?

At the outset this was clearly an exterior pattern of disease, but that was two months ago. Now the symptoms involve a fever with no aversion to cold, thus the pattern is strictly one of the interior.

2. Is the cough caused by heat or cold?

The sputum is of major significance in determining whether a cough is hot or cold in nature. The cold type of cough manifests in clear, white sputum, whereas the heat type produces thick, yellow sputum. The patient's history reveals that the original cold pattern has transformed into a pattern of heat. The sputum, originally white, is now thick and yellow. In addition, analysis of all the other symptoms confirms that the pattern is one of heat.

3. Is there a deficiency of Spleen qi?

There are indeed symptoms commonly associated with Spleen qi deficiency, such as poor appetite and abdominal distention, but in this case these symptoms are not related to a deficiency of Spleen qi. Rather they are the consequence of severe heat injuring the body fluids. The stools have become dry and slow, leading to obstruction of the qi in the Large Intestine. This in turn has influenced the function of the Stomach and Spleen and resulted in the above symptoms. The symptoms themselves, however, are not evidence of Spleen qi deficiency.

Conclusion

1. According to the eight principles:
   Interior, heat, excess.

2. According to etiology diagnosis:
   Phlegm-heat.

3. According to Organ diagnosis:
   Phlegm-heat in the Lung.

Treatment principle

1. Remove the phlegm.
2. Clear the heat.
3. Regulate the Lung qi.

Selection of points

LI-11 *(qu chi)* through to L-5 *(chi ze)*
L-10 *(yu ji)*
S-40 *(feng long)*
GV-14 *(da zhui)*
CV-17 *(shan zhong)*

Explanation of points

LI-11 *(qu chi)* is the sea point of the hand yang brightness channel. It is a very important point for removing heat and regulating the qi and blood.

L-5 *(chi ze)* is the sea point of the hand greater yin channel. This point has a strong effect in eliminating heat from the Lung and regulating the directional flow of Lung qi. Thus it is commonly used in treating heat or phlegm-heat resulting in cough, asthma, and hemoptysis (coughing with blood).

The Lung and Large Intestine have an interior-exterior relationship and both of the above points are sea points. They are also close to one another and possess a similar therapeutic function, the removal of heat. The threading method is utilized for two reasons: it requires less needles, and it is a very safe way to puncture L-5.

L-10 *(yu ji)* is the spring point of the hand greater yin channel, and has a good effect in removing heat, alleviating pain, and removing obstruction from the channel. It is therefore chosen to treat the pain in the larynx or pharynx, chest, and upper back.

S-40 *(feng long)* is the most important point on the body for removing phlegm; it also acts to remove dampness.

GV-14 *(da zhui)* is indicated here for the removal of heat. The point is rapidly punctured before the main treatment begins. Then the patient lies on her back for the remainder of the treatment.

CV-17 *(shan zhong)* is the influential point of qi. It is very effective in regulating the directional flow of qi both locally and generally throughout the body. This point is commonly used for stagnation and reversal of qi in both the chest and the epigastric region.

Follow-up

After two daily treatments the patient's temperature was between 38 and 38.5ºC. On the fourth day her temperature remained below 38ºC, but the cough became worse with a lot of sputum. Two more points, CV-12 *(zhong wan)* and LI-4 *(he gu)*, were added to the prescription, and the patient was treated every day for a week. The cough was then very mild and there was no sputum. She had two further treatments during the next week, and also took the Chinese herbs listed below for two weeks. Thereafter she was symptom free.

Cortex Mori Albae *(sang bai pi)*
Semen Pruni Armeniacae *(xing ren)*
Radix Platycodi Grandiflorum *(jie geng)*
Semen Coicis Lachryma jobi *(yi yi ren)*
Cortex Lycii Radicis *(di gu pi)*
Sclerotium Poriae Cocos *(fu ling)*

Herba Lophatheri Gracilis *(dan zhu ye)*
Fructus Trichosanthis *(gua lou)*
Pericarpium Citri Reticulatae *(chen pi)*
Rhizoma Pinelliae Ternatae *(ban xia)*
Radix Scutellariae Baicalensis *(huang qin)*
Radix Glycyrrhizae Uralensis *(gan cao)*

CASE 6: **Female, age 60**

Main complaint

Cough

History

The patient has a recurrent cough of four years' duration. Last week the symptoms returned.

Four years ago bronchitis was diagnosed, the main symptom being a non-asthmatic cough, onset normally in the winter or when the patient catches cold. One week ago after exposure to cold the symptoms returned. The main symptoms are severe cough, worse during the night, and the patient can only sleep 3-4 hours per night. There is excessive white sputum, the patient has a feeling of being cold without a fever, and there is a stifling sensation in the chest. She has a poor appetite and loose stools, with 4-5 bowel movements per day.

Tongue	Light red body, white, greasy coating
Pulse	Thin, slippery
Analysis of symptoms	1. Four-year history of cough—Lung qi deficiency.
	2. Excessive white sputum—retention of phlegm-dampness in the Lung.
	3. Stifling sensation in the chest—stagnation of qi.
	4. Feeling of being cold—yang deficiency.
	5. Poor appetite and loose stools—Spleen qi deficiency.
	6. White, greasy tongue coating, slippery pulse—phlegm and dampness.

Basic theory of case

The Lung and Spleen have a close physiological relationship such that if one Organ becomes diseased it will often influence the other. According to the five phase theory the Spleen is earth and the Lung is metal, and thus they have an inter-promoting or mother-son relationship. According to Organ theory the Lung governs the qi of the body and the Spleen is the source of qi and blood. These two Organs are both involved in the production and distribution of acquired ('post-heaven') qi, as distinct from vital essence or congenital ('pre-heaven') qi.

The Spleen and Stomach produce essence and qi by a process of extracting the nutritive materials from food and liquids. The Lung distributes the essence and qi to different parts of the body in order to replenish what has been depleted by the normal demands of the body's daily activities.

When the Spleen qi is deficient the transformation and transportation of food and liquid is impaired, which reduces the amount of qi and food essence. The various tissues and Organs of the body will thus become malnourished. The Lung qi often becomes deficient as a consequence of Spleen qi deficiency. Conversely, when the Lung qi becomes deficient it may divert the food essence and qi of the Stomach and Spleen upwards to the Lungs in order to maintain a reasonable metabolic rate. If allowed to persist, this abnormal condition will cause Spleen qi deficiency.

In the clinic, Lung and Spleen qi deficiency often occur together. For example, lecturers who give long speeches and therefore consume Lung qi often lose their appetites. The longer the speech, the greater the loss of Lung qi and thus the loss of appetite, as Spleen function is affected. Similarly, when there is Spleen qi deficiency the general energy level is not good, and this will often lead to shortness of breath.

Cause of disease

Phlegm-dampness

The manifestations in this case mainly involve cough with excessive white sputum, and the tongue coating is white and greasy. Both of these symptoms indicate the retention of phlegm and dampness.

Site of disease

Lung and Spleen

There are three main symptoms of a Lung disorder: stifling sensation in the chest, recurrent cough, and excessive sputum.

The poor appetite and loose stools indicate a Spleen disorder.

Pathological change

The Lung is responsible for respiration and for the distribution of protective qi to the surface of the body. The protective qi protects the body from invasion by pathogenic factors. This patient's recurrent cough has consumed the Lung qi, which in turn has weakened the protective qi. The body's resistance is accordingly diminished, which has made it easier for pathogenic factors to penetrate the superficial tissues. The greater the decline in Lung qi, the easier it is for pathogenic factors to invade the body, and the more the pathogenic factors invade, the worse the level of Lung qi deficiency. A self-weakening cycle is therefore established: after the invasion by pathogenic cold, the Lung's inability to disperse and descend becomes worse, leading to recurrence of cough.

The patient is suffering from qi deficiency. Qi is strongly influenced by the environment. The yang is dominant during the day, at which time the qi receives support from the environment. At night the yang in the environment is weak; the deficiency of qi is then more obvious, and the cough becomes worse.

The Lung is involved in the process of the body's water metabolism. When the Lung qi is weak, the distribution of fluids to the rest of the body is interrupted, and this leads to an accumulation of body fluids, which is harmful to the body.

There are four types of harmful body fluids: 1. retention of dampness; 2. congested fluids; 3. retention of pathogenic water (edema); and 4. phlegm.

In this case the harmful body fluid is phlegm. Phlegm blocks the normal passage of qi in the Lungs and causes a stifling sensation in the chest. Chronic Lung qi deficiency can lead to Spleen qi deficiency in which symptoms of poor appetite and loose stools develop. The patient also has a feeling of being cold, which implies a deficiency of yang. The yang deficiency is associated with the qi deficiency, thus we conclude that the patient suffers from Spleen yang deficiency.

The white, greasy tongue coating and slippery pulse clearly indicate an accumulation of phlegm-dampness. The thin pulse is an indication of deficiency.

Another way of explaining this case is that the deficiency of Spleen yang (earth) impaired its ability to nourish the Lung qi (metal) which in turn became deficient. The symptoms are identical.

The key to diagnosing this patient is found in the history of her illness. The history reveals that she developed chronic Lung qi deficiency which eventually led to Spleen yang deficiency.

Fig. 2

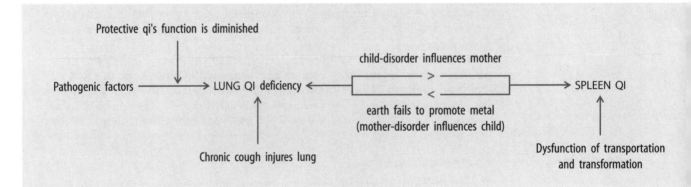

Pattern of disease

The patient has severe cough with no aversion to cold, indicating an interior pattern.

The white sputum, feeling of cold, and white tongue coating indicate a cold pattern.

The long history of recurrent cough and the ease with which she catches cold, poor appetite, and loose stools indicate a pattern of deficiency.

The patient now has a severe cough with excessive sputum and a stifling sensation in the chest. These symptoms form a pattern of excess (retention of phlegm).

Additional notes

1. Does the exterior pattern remain?

The patient's illness was initially caused by exposure to cold, an external pathogenic factor, but she now has only a feeling of being cold, with no aversion to cold. The cough is the main complaint and the site of the disease is now in the Lung. It is thus an interior pattern, and no longer exterior.

2. How do we judge the excess and deficiency in this case?

The patient has Spleen and Lung qi deficiency complicated by retention of phlegm-dampness, which is an excessive disorder. There is thus a mixture or combination of excess and deficiency. In the clinic the patient presented with a very severe cough and profuse, white sputum. She coughed but had no wheezing and there were no symptoms to suggest severe Lung qi deficiency this time, such as weak cough or voice, or shortness of breath. Although the patient had symptoms of Spleen yang deficiency, they were not the reason she came for treatment. The diagnosis should be made according to the main complaint, and therefore the excessive pattern is the main problem here.

3. Is there a Heart disorder in this case?

Insomnia can be caused by a disturbance of the spirit. In this case sleep is being disturbed by the severe cough rather than the pathogenic factors attacking the spirit or Heart directly, and thus there is no Heart disorder.

Conclusion

1. According to the eight principles:
   Interior, cold, mixture of deficiency and excess (deficiency within excess).
2. According to etiology diagnosis:
   Phlegm-dampness.
3. According to Organ diagnosis:
   Retention of phlegm-dampness in the Lung. Lung qi deficiency and Spleen yang deficiency.

Treatment principle

1. Eliminate the phlegm and regulate the dispersing function of the Lung.
2. Warm and reinforce the Lung and Spleen.

Selection of points

S-13 *(qi hu)*
CV-13 *(shang wan)*
L-7 *(lie que)*
S-40 *(feng long)* on one side
S-36 *(zu san li)* on one side

Explanation of points

S-13 *(qi hu)* is located in the upper burner in close proximity to the top of the Lung. It regulates the dispersing function and directional flow of the Lung qi, and also removes any obstruction from the channel. It is therefore used to relieve chest pain. In the clinic this point has many indications including a stifling sensation in the chest, wheezing, chest pain, and reversal of qi.

CV-13 *(shang wan)* is the meeting point of the conception vessel with foot yang brightness and hand greater yang, and is located in the upper part of the middle burner, close to the upper burner. Thus, in addition to its effect on the middle burner, it also has a strong effect on disorders of the upper burner. It regulates and mildly tonifies the qi. It is also useful for correcting the directional flow of the Lung qi, resolving phlegm, and calming the spirit. It is a good choice in this case to deal with the severe cough with excessive sputum which disrupts the patient's sleep.

L-7 *(lie que)* is the connecting point of the hand greater yin and is indicated for promoting the Lung qi and expelling the pathogenic factors.

S-40 *(feng long)* is the connecting point of the foot yang brightness and is very effective in removing phlegm. Phlegm may develop when the metabolism of the middle burner is weakened. This point corrects the weakness and promotes the removal of phlegm from the body.

S-36 *(zu san li)* is one of the most important points for tonification, both for the middle burner and the general condition. It is indicated when there is phlegm, congested fluids, or dampness caused by qi or yang deficiency.

Combination of points	S-40 *(feng long)* and S-36 *(zu san li)* are punctured unilaterally in order to reduce the number of points used. In this case their combined functions of tonifying qi and removing phlegm are very useful. It does not matter which point is needled on which side.
	S-13 *(qi hu)* and CV-13 *(shang wan)* both act on the Lungs. One is located on the upper aspect and the other on the lower aspect. Their combined effect corrects the directional flow of qi and regulates the dispersing function of the Lung. They are thus a good pair for alleviating cough and pain.
Follow-up	After one treatment the cough was much better and the patient was sleeping well. She was treated three more times on alternate days, after which the cough and sputum were almost gone. The treatment principle then changed to one of tonifying the Spleen and Lung, twice a week for four weeks, using the points listed below. After this the patient only coughed occasionally and treatment was ended.
	CV-11 *(jian li)* S-36 *(zu san li)* L-7 *(lie que)* or L-9 *(tai yuan)*

CASE 7: **Male, age 40**

Main complaint	Cough
History	The patient complained that since yesterday he has suffered from very severe bouts of coughing of a choking character. The cough is immediately followed by wheezing and a distending sensation which radiates upwards from the Lung. The cough causes chest and hypochondriac pain, and the cough becomes more severe when he lies flat on the bed. When he coughs he brings up thick sputum, sometimes containing a small quantity of blood clots. He is thirsty, likes to drink, and has a bitter taste in the mouth. The other symptoms include poor appetite, general lassitude, yellow urine, constipation for two days, and a hot feeling on the skin over the entire body.
Tongue	Red body, yellow coating
Pulse	Surging and forceful. The right distal region is stronger.
Analysis of symptoms	1. Episodic and sharp projective-like cough with a choking quality, followed by wheezing with a distending sensation radiating upwards— fire attacking the Lung. 2. Sticky, thick, blood-tinged sputum—phlegm-heat. 3. Chest and hypochondriac pain caused by severe cough, bitter taste in the mouth—Liver fire. 4. Thirsty, likes to drink, yellow urine, and constipation—heat. 5. General lassitude, poor appetite—qi deficiency. 6. Hot feeling on the body surface, red tongue, yellow coating, surging and forceful pulse—heat.
Basic theory of case	A central concept in Chinese medicine is to view the body as an integral whole. Each of the Organs has its own group of functions, and the interrelationship among all of the Organs is the foundation of good health. A discussion of the relationship between the Lungs and Liver will be useful in the context of this case. The Lung governs the overall qi of the body by causing it to disperse and descend. The Liver is responsible for the free-flow of qi. The Chinese term for this Liver function is *shū xiè*. *Shū* means to transport smoothly

and efficiently, *xiè* to travel upwards and outwards, like bulbs growing in the springtime.

We know that both of these Organs are involved in activities relating to the qi, particularly in ascending and descending. The Lung is located in the body at a higher level than any of the other yin Organs. The function of the Lung qi is primarily one of causing the qi to descend. The Liver is associated with the spring, wind, and wood. These three aspects paint a natural picture of the Liver, the activity of its qi primarily being one of ascending and opening out.

When the Lung is attacked by pathogenic factors its descending function is impaired, which may result in a reversal in the direction of its qi, leading to cough. When the Liver qi over-ascends and extends, it may either cause or aggravate this reversal of the Lung qi.

Cause of disease

Pathogenic fire

Fire is a yang pathogenic factor characterized by a tendency to ascend rapidly. Symptoms associated with fire reflect this characteristic and tend to appear suddenly, severely, and on the upper aspect of the body.

This patient's severe cough appeared suddenly and produced a loud, whoops-like sound, followed immediately by wheezing and a distending sensation which radiated upwards from the Lung. This type of severe reversal in the direction of the Lung qi is caused by an attack of pathogenic fire.

Site of disease

Lung and Liver

The patient has a cough, blood-tinged sputum, and wheezing, all of which indicate the involvement of the Lung.

The cough has led to chest, intercostal, and hypochondriac pain, involving the Liver.

Pathological change

Under normal conditions we know that the Lung qi descends and the Liver qi ascends. The qi is associated with yang; over-ascending of Liver qi will give rise to pathogenic fire. This Liver fire spurts upwards through the channels and attacks the Lungs, suddenly reversing the direction of its qi. The episodic cough had a rapid onset and caused a distending sensation which migrated upwards and was followed by wheezing, indicating that internal pathogenic fire is the cause of the disease.

Fire consumes the body fluids and injures the vessels of the Lung, resulting in thick, sticky sputum with bloody clots. The Liver fire rises up and disturbs the distribution of qi and blood. This impairs the qi circulation in the Lung and chest, leading to stagnation and pain.

When the patient lies down the cough becomes worse because qi circulation is made more difficult. The bitter taste in the mouth is produced by the heat from the fire which has 'steamed' the bile of the Gallbladder. The fire consumes the body fluids and causes constipation, yellow urine, thirst, and a hot feeling on the surface of the body.

The red tongue with a yellow coating, and the surging, forceful pulse reflect the strong internal heat. The first position on the right wrist represents the Lung, and the pulse is stronger here than in all the other positions, indicating that Liver fire is attacking the Lung. The Lung is associated with metal and the Liver with wood. The Liver fire attacks the Lung, thus wood counteracts metal. In Chinese medicine this is a very important concept known as 'wood fire scorching and torturing metal'. *See Fig. 3.*

Pattern of disease

The site of the disease is the Lung and the Liver, indicating an interior pattern.

The thick, sticky sputum, hot sensation, thirst, yellow urine, and constipation are all symptoms of heat.

Since the disease was caused by pathogenic fire, the pattern is one of excess.

Fig. 3

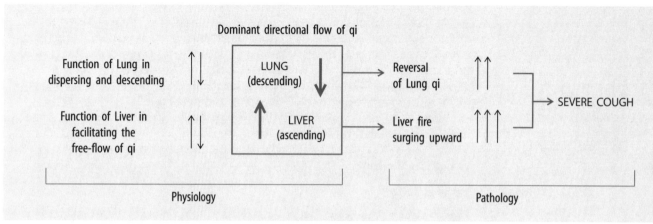

Additional notes

1. Is there any deficiency of qi?

This patient experiences general lassitude and a poor appetite, which reflect the injury to the qi. This is caused by fire consuming the energy of the body. The excessive heat produced by the hyperactivity of yang consumes and injures the qi. *The Inner Classic* describes this phenomenon as 'fire devouring qi.' Thus in this case the qi was not initially deficient, but has become injured.

2. How does one determine whether the cough is caused by heat in the Lung or by Liver fire scorching the Lung?

These two patterns can exhibit identical symptoms, e.g., cough with yellow sputum, hot sensation on the body, thirst, red tongue, yellow coating, and rapid pulse. The distinguishing characteristics are as follows:

i. Cough caused by wood (Liver) counteracting metal (Lung) is episodic with a choking quality. Usually the cough is very severe, incessant, and leaves the patient breathless. For a short time after the coughing fit the patient will often have a red face and red eyes caused by an inability to breathe during the coughing fit.

   Lung-heat cough may also be strong but its pattern does not exhibit the clear bouts of incessant coughing which cause red eyes and facial complexion.

ii. When Liver fire invades the Lung the nature of the pain is different because it extends to the hypochondriac region.

   Heat in the Lung will usually only cause chest pain.

iii. Cough from Liver fire is usually sudden. There may be a reason for the onset, e.g., emotional change or insufficient rest, but there will not be any history or evidence of invasion by pathogenic factors.

   Lung-heat cough usually has a slower onset and a history of exposure to some pathogenic factor. The symptoms of Lung-heat cough will appear from one to several days after exposure.

Conclusion

1. According to the eight principles:
   Interior, heat, excessive.
2. According to etiology diagnosis:
   Pathogenic fire.
3. According to Organ diagnosis:
   Liver fire scorching the Lung.

Treatment principle

1. Sedate the Liver fire.

2. Remove the Lung heat.

3. Stop the coughing.

Selection of points

CV-22 *(tian tu)*
S-25 *(tian shu)*
L-6 *(kong zui)* on one side
L-5 *(chi ze)* on one side
G-34 *(yang ling quan)*
Liv-2 *(xing jian)*

Explanation of points

CV-22 *(tian tu)* regulates the dispersing function of Lung qi and corrects the reversal of qi. It is effective in treating the distending sensation which radiates upwards, and also for removing heat.

S-25 *(tian shu)* is the alarm point of the Large Intestine and is a very good point for removing obstruction and regulating the qi of the Large Intestine. In this case the patient has constipation; evacuating the stool from the hand yang brightness Organ will help to remove heat from the metal phase (Lung and Large Intestine) in general.

L-6 *(kong zui)* is the accumulating point of the Lung channel. It is effective in regulating the descending function of the Lung, removing heat, and stopping hemorrhage. It is a good choice here for treating the sputum with bloody clots. The point also removes obstruction and relieves pain in the chest.

L-5 *(chi ze)* is the sea point of the hand greater yin. It removes heat from the blood level. The three-edge (triangular) needle can be used here to draw heat from the blood.

G-34 *(yang ling quan)* is the sea point of the Gallbladder channel. This point is indicated for the regulation of Liver and Gallbladder qi. It also removes heat and dampness.

Liv-2 *(xing jian)*, the spring point of the Liver channel, is very effective for removing Liver fire and obstruction from the Liver channel.

Combination of points

L-6 *(kong zui)* and L-5 *(chi ze)*, the accumulating point and the sea point of the Lung channel respectively, are used in treating acute problems, especially at the blood level. In this case they are chosen to stop hemorrhage and eliminate fire.

G-34 *(yang ling quan)* and Liv-2 *(xing jian)* are combined to remove heat from the Gallbladder and Liver, one point from the yang channel and the other from the yin channel. One is a spring point and the other a sea point. They are a strong combination for removing heat.

Follow-up

This patient was treated each day for three days. The cough, chest pain, and hypochondriac pain disappeared and the sputum was no longer blood-stained. At this point he still had an occasional dry cough, felt irritable, and had dream-disturbed sleep and dry stools, thus the internal heat remained strong. He was therefore treated with Antelope Horn Pill to Clear the Lungs *(ling yang qing fei wan)* and Cattle Gallstone Pill to Clear Fire *(niu huang qing huo wan)* for a week, after which he felt fine.

CASE 8: **Female, age 41**

Main complaint

Cough

History

This patient has had a recurrent cough for over two years. When it recurs it can be either mild or severe. The cough is accompanied by thick, yellow, sticky sputum which is both scanty in quantity and difficult to bring up. The patient is thirsty and has a dry, hoarse throat. She has a feeble voice, poor appetite, and prefers not to speak.

In the afternoon she develops a slight fever (37.5°C- 37.8°C). She also has a malar flush, night sweats, and dream-disturbed sleep. In addition, there is a history of lower back pain and soreness and weakness of the lower limbs. Over the past six months there has been no menstruation.

Tongue	Deep red tongue body, very thin tongue coating
Pulse	Thin, rapid

Analysis of symptoms

1. Chronic cough, thick, sticky, and yellow sputum which is scanty and difficult to expectorate—Lung yin deficiency.
2. Feeble voice, avoids speaking, poor appetite—qi deficiency.
3. Lower back pain, soreness and weakness of the lower limbs— Kidney yin deficiency.
4. Dryness of the mouth and throat, afternoon fevers, night sweats, dream-disturbed sleep, malar flush—yin deficiency.
5. Amenorrhea—malnourishment of the blood or deficiency of the sea of blood (penetrating vessel).
6. Deep red tongue, very thin coating, thin, rapid pulse—yin deficiency.

Basic theory of case

The Lung is located in the upper burner and has the function of dispersing and descending. This includes the dispersal of food essence from the Spleen to the various Organs, including the Kidney, and also to the various body tissues. This function replenishes the stock of food essence consumed by the body during its daily activities.

The Kidney is located in the lower burner and has the function of storing the vital essence. The stored essence is both congenital ('pre-heaven') and acquired ('post-heaven'). Essence is associated with yin. The Kidney essence is transformed into Kidney yin which nourishes the yin of all the Organs. As such it is known as the root of the body's yin.

The Kidney yin nourishes all of the Organs, supporting their physiological functions. Thus both the Lung and Kidney are involved in the general nourishment of the body. According to five phase theory the Lung is associated with metal and the Kidney with water. The relationship is thus inter-promoting, or one of mother and son. The emphasis in this relationship is directed towards the interaction of yin and body fluids.

Fig. 4

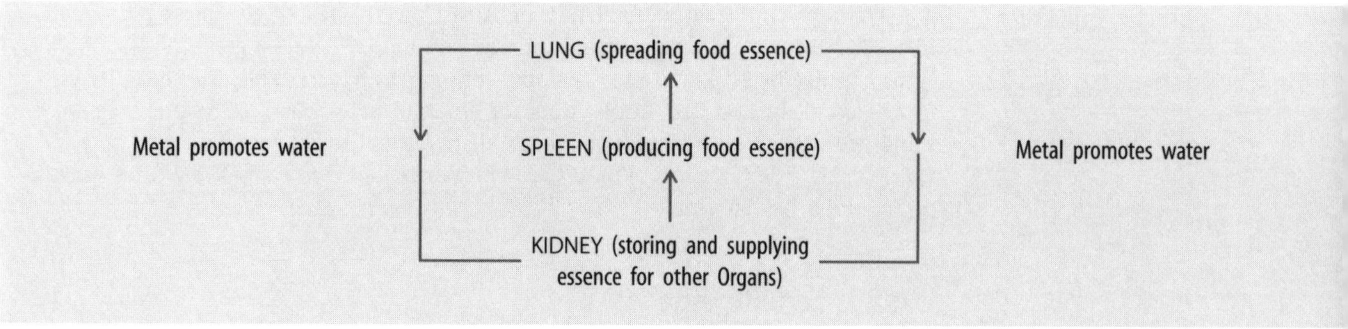

LUNG (spreading food essence)

Metal promotes water   SPLEEN (producing food essence)   Metal promotes water

KIDNEY (storing and supplying essence for other Organs)

Cause of disease

Yin deficiency

The patient has a chronic cough of two-years' duration. In addition there is thick, yellow, and sticky sputum which is scanty and difficult to expectorate; dryness of the throat, night sweats, and afternoon fevers. This group of symptoms indicates malnourishment of the body due to yin deficiency, and also deficiency of body fluids.

Site of disease

Lung and Kidney

The cough, dryness in the throat, and hoarseness are the main evidence of a Lung disorder.

The lower back pain, soreness and weakness of the lower limbs suggest a disorder of the Kidney.

Pathological change

All of the Organs and tissues of the body have a yang-qi aspect and a yin-fluid aspect. A patient with chronic cough may have an injury to either the Lung qi or yin, but in the clinic these two aspects display separate symptom patterns.

This patient has had a recurrent cough for over two years. The characteristics in this case, such as the scanty, yellow, sticky, and thick sputum which is difficult to expectorate, point to an injury of the Lung yin. There is deficiency of the yin and body fluids which causes malnourishment of the Lung, and in turn impairs the Lung's function of dispersing and descending. The combination of these factors makes recovery a slow and difficult process.

The throat is regarded as the gateway to the voice and the entrance to the Lung. Lung yin deficiency automatically leads to malnourishment of the throat, dryness in the mouth and throat, and hoarseness. Because the body fluids are deficient, the sputum is scanty and difficult to expectorate.

The yin and yang of the body will always try to balance and control one another. When one becomes deficient it will cause a preponderance of the other. The yin deficiency creates a preponderance of yang, which in turn causes heat symptoms in the body. This internal heat is caused by yin deficiency and is thus a false or 'empty' heat (also known as heat from deficiency). Such heat leads to afternoon fevers and 'steams' the resurgence of body fluids in the form of night sweats. The heat rises up to disturb the spirit. The disturbance of the spirit in turn causes dream-disturbed sleep. Another obvious symptom of yin-deficient heat rising to the head is the malar flush.

In this case there is chronic Lung yin deficiency, which over a period of time has attacked the yin of the Kidney because the metal (Lung) is unable to support the water (Kidney). The lower back is the dwelling of the Kidney, and the Kidney also controls the bones. Kidney yin deficiency results in malnourishment of the knee joints and lower back, and this explains the lower back pain and soreness and weakness of the lower limbs.

Menstrual blood is part of the body's yin. Since the yin is deficient the penetrating and conception vessels are not adequately filled, resulting in amenorrhea. Both the deep red tongue with very thin coating and the thin, rapid pulse indicate a pattern of yin-deficient heat.

Pattern of disease

This patient has a two-year history of cough and afternoon fevers with no aversion to cold, indicating an interior pattern of disease.

The yellow, sticky, thick sputum accompanied by afternoon fevers, dryness in the mouth, sore throat, night sweats, deep red tongue, and rapid pulse indicate a pattern of heat.

The soreness, weakness of the lower back and knee joints, thin pulse, and empty heat symptoms indicate a pattern of deficiency.

Additional notes

1. How does one distinguish excessive from deficient heat in the Lung?

The retention of phlegm-heat in the Lung is an excessive heat pattern. The heat from deficiency pattern may involve just the Lung yin deficiency, or the Lung and Kidney yin deficiency combined. Both types may display cough and yellow sputum. The distinguishing characteristics include the quantity of sputum, the nature of the heat, and the quality of the tongue and pulse.

i. When there is retention of phlegm and heat in the Lung, there will be a large quantity of yellow sputum.

When the Lung yin is deficient, the sputum will be scanty. There may also be a dry cough with no sputum.

ii. The excessive pattern of heat will manifest in a red complexion. There will be thirst with a preference for cold drinks, yellow urine, and constipation.

The empty or deficient pattern of heat causes a malar flush, night sweats, and burning in the five centers. There will also be thirst, but usually the patient will prefer not to drink much. Various types of low grade fever may emerge, like tidal fevers or afternoon fevers.

iii. The excessive phlegm-heat pattern will manifest clearly on the tongue in the form of a thick, yellow, and greasy tongue coating. The pulse will generally be slippery, rapid, and forceful.

In the case of Lung yin deficiency, the sputum is scanty and thus there will be little evidence of phlegm on the tongue coating. The coating may be thin and yellow, or there may be very little tongue coating at all. The pulse is thin, rapid, and forceless.

2. Is there any qi deficiency in this case?

This patient has a feeble voice and a tendency to avoid talking. She also has a poor appetite. These symptoms indicate a deficiency of qi.

Yin and yang have a mutually interdependent relationship. Yang helps in the creation of yin and vice versa. When there is yin deficiency the foundation of yang becomes weak. In this case, the symptoms of qi deficiency result from a chronic deficiency of yin. In diagnosing this case one cannot conclude that there is only deficiency of qi, because the qi deficiency itself has been caused by chronic yin deficiency.

In the previous case (number 7) there were also symptoms of qi deficiency; however these were caused by excessively strong heat. There are many causes for symptoms of qi deficiency and it is thus very important to consider each case carefully.

3. How does one distinguish the cough caused by Lung yin deficiency from that caused by Lung and Kidney yin deficiency combined?

Both of these patterns involve a cough that can be entirely dry or produce scanty amounts of sputum. They may also display many symptoms of heat from deficiency. The key to distinguishing these patterns is to see whether the patient has the symptoms which suggest Kidney yin deficiency, e.g., whether there is soreness and weakness of the lower back, and nocturnal emissions in men. If there are no Kidney symptoms present, then the Kidney is not involved.

Conclusion

1. According to the eight principles:
   Interior, heat, deficiency.
2. According to Organ diagnosis:
   Deficiency of Lung and Kidney yin.

Treatment principle

Nourish and tonify the Lung and Kidney yin.

Selection of points

B-13 *(fei shu)*
B-17 *(ge shu)*
B-20 *(pi shu)*
B-23 *(shen shu)*
L-7 *(lie que)*
K-6 *(zhao hai)*

Explanation of points

In Chinese *shū* means to remove or make smooth passage. The associated *(shu)* points of the back are very effective in both regulating and tonifying the qi of the yin and yang Organs. The yang Organs have different characteristics from the yin Organs. The yin Organs are solid; they store and process the body's nutrients. For example, the Liver stores the blood and the Kidney stores vital essence. The yang Organs are hollow and normally keep themselves functioning properly by allowing substances to pass through without being retained. The yin Organs have problems of deficiency rather than excess, while the yang Organs tend to have problems with excess rather than deficiency. The associated points are commonly used in treating deficiency patterns in the yin Organs.

The associated points are usually punctured in groups of three, four, or more. Many of the associated points are considered dangerous due to their proximity to the lung. Because of their precarious location only limited stimulation of the points is advised. The points are chosen according to the result of the practitioner's diagnosis. Here the purpose is to nourish the Kidney, Lung, and blood.

B-13 *(fei shu)* is a good point for nourishing the Lung yin and reinforcing the Lung qi.

B-17 *(ge shu)* is located at the juncture of the upper and middle burners. It is used to regulate the qi of both the upper and middle burners. It can thus support B-13 *(fei shu)* in restoring the directional flow of qi. B-17 *(ge shu)* is the influential point of the blood, and many kinds of blood disorders are treated with this point, including amenorrhea. It is very effective in nourishing the yin and clearing deficiency-type heat patterns, and is also indicated for reducing the fever and relieving the night sweats.

B-20 *(pi shu)* is used to tonify the Spleen. A healthy Spleen will support the function of the Kidney and Lung.

B-23 *(shen shu)* is used to tonify the Kidney.

L-7 *(lie que)* is the confluent point of the conception vessel, which influences many menstrual disorders and is connected to the Kidney. When both the Lung and Kidney are affected, L-7 *(lie que)* is particularly indicated.

K-6 *(zhao hai)* is the confluent point of the yin-heel vessel. The main functions of this point include clearing the heat, nourishing the yin, soothing the throat, and calming the spirit.

Combination of points

L-7 *(lie que)* and K-6 *(zhao hai)* regulate the Lung qi and nourish the Lung and Kidney yin. This combination is good for relaxing the diaphragm, soothing the throat, and stopping cough or wheezing.

Follow-up

This patient was treated on alternate days for two weeks, after which her temperature was normal and the night sweats and afternoon fevers had disappeared. The cough gradually improved but was still present. She then continued treatments for three months consisting of ten treatments every four weeks, followed by a one-week break. The symptoms gradually disappeared and she was discharged.

Diagnostic principles for cough

1. Diagnosis of cough according to etiology and pathological change

i. Cough may be caused by an invasion of the body by any of the six external pathogenic factors. Irrespective of which pathogenic factor is involved, or whether the skin or the mouth and nose is attacked, the pathological change always causes dysfunction of the Lung qi in dispersing and descending. In the eight-principle differentiation, this is a pattern of excess.

ii. Cough may also be caused by internal disorders. Either there is no obvious external pathogenic factor involved, or the disease has reached a stage where the original invasion has disappeared and only an interior disorder remains. Examples would include retention of phlegm, deficiency of Lung qi, or Liver fire attacking the Lung. No matter what the underlying cause, the Lung's function in both dispersing and descending is affected, leading to cough. In the eight-principle differentiation, the pattern may be excessive, deficient, or a combination of both.

Fig. 5

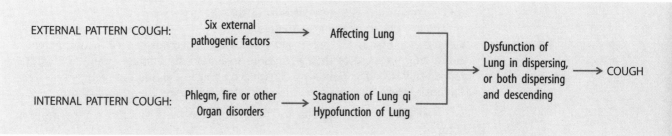

Fig. 6   2. Differential diagnosis of cough

MAIN SYMPTOMS			ACCOMPANYING SYMPTOMS	

1. Exterior patterns:

Wind-cold type:	COUGH	White and clear sputum	Exterior cold symptoms:	Aversion to cold and fever, no sweating, thin white tongue coating, floating and tight pulse
Wind-heat type:	COUGH	Yellow and sticky sputum	Exterior heat symptoms:	Fever, slight aversion to cold, sweating, sore throat, yellow tongue coating, floating and rapid pulse
Dryness type:	COUGH	Scanty sputum, difficult to expectorate	Exterior dryness symptoms:	Slight aversion to cold and slight fever, dry nose and throat

2. Interior patterns:

Retention of phlegm in Lung	COUGH	Excessive white and clear sputum	Symptoms involve dampness:	Stifling sensation in the chest, heaviness around the body, poor appetite, etc.
Phlegm-heat in Lung	COUGH	Excessive yellow and sticky sputum	Symptoms involve heat:	Chest pain, fever or hot sensations, thirsty, etc.
Liver fire scorching Lung	COUGH	Severe choking cough with yellow and sticky sputum	Symptoms involve Liver fire:	Intercoastal and hypochondriac pain, irritability, insomnia, etc.
Lung qi deficiency	COUGH	Excessive white and clear sputum	Symptoms involve qi deficiency:	Shortness of breath, weak voice, general lassitude, etc.
Lung yin deficiency	COUGH	No sputum or scanty and sticky sputum or sputum streaked with blood	Symptoms involve yin deficiency:	Tidal fever, night sweats, dry mouth, etc.

3. Entire diagnostic procedure for cough

This procedure mainly follows the eight-principle theory of diagnosis whereby one distinguishes whether a pattern is interior or exterior, deficient or excessive, and cold or heat:

i.   In order to determine whether the pattern is exterior or interior, one must ascertain whether the patient has a fever and an aversion to cold.
ii. If there is hypofunction of the Organs or a deficiency of qi or blood, the pattern is deficient. If the pathogenic factors are strong or retained within the body, the pattern is one of excess.
iii. Heat or cold patterns are distinguished by the color and quality of the phlegm.

Fig. 7   The entire diagnostic procedure for cough is summarized in the following chart.

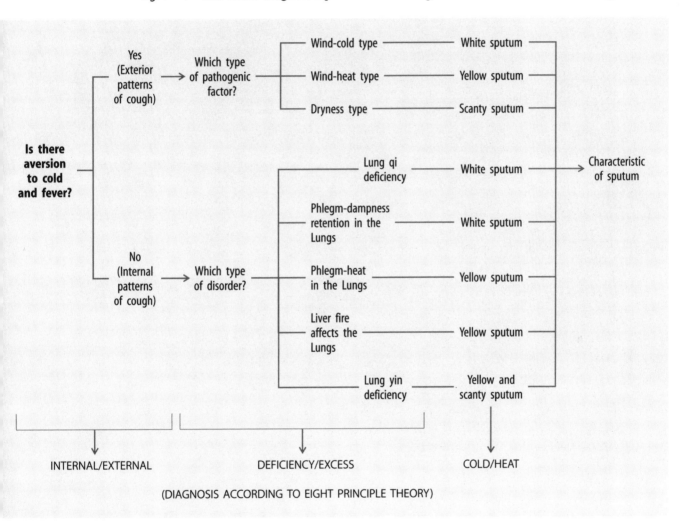

(DIAGNOSIS ACCORDING TO EIGHT PRINCIPLE THEORY)

Dizziness

CASE 9: **Female, age 63**

Main complaint

Drowsiness and dizziness

History

The patient's symptoms first began two months ago. They were episodic and mild in nature, and were occasionally accompanied by slight, lateral headaches. She had no idea as to the cause of her condition, which did not deteriorate over the two month period.

One week ago, after an emotional upset, the dizziness, headache, and drowsiness all became worse. The other main symptoms in this case were dream-disturbed sleep, palpitations, general lassitude, and distention in the intercostal, hypochondriac, epigastric, and abdominal regions. The patient has a poor appetite and bitter taste in the mouth. She does not complain of being thirsty. She has a dry stool every other day. Urination is normal.

Tongue

Dark pale body; thick, greasy, slightly yellow coating

Pulse

Wiry, slippery, and slightly rapid

Analysis of symptoms

1. Dizziness, headache, drowsiness—failure of the clear yang to rise.
2. General lassitude, abdominal and epigastric distention—
   loss of Spleen function in transportation and transformation.
3. Palpitations, dream-disturbed sleep—spirit disturbance.
4. Intercostal and hypochondriac region distention—stagnation of Liver qi.
5. Bitter taste in the mouth, dry stools—retention of heat.
6. Pale dark tongue—qi and blood deficiency, poor circulation.
7. Thick, greasy and slightly yellow tongue coating, slippery, rapid pulse—
   damp-heat.
8. Wiry pulse—stagnation of Liver qi.

Basic theory of case

Dizziness is a subjective symptom of feeling like the environment is moving or shaking. When a person feels as if they or the room is spinning, it is called vertigo. In Chinese medicine, the word 'dizziness' is used to describe both these conditions. In mild cases the patient feels only some discomfort when moving the head or experiences episodic darkness before the eyes. In severe cases the patient loses his or her balance and has to lie down. This symptom can be accompanied by nausea and vomiting. Clinically, dizziness and vertigo can be the main complaint or just a secondary symptom. Remember that in traditional Chinese medicine these symptoms are often associated with dysfunction of the internal Organs; they should not be considered a local symptom of the head.

The yang qi is clear, clean, and lightweight in nature, and has a tendency to ascend. The clear yang rises to the highest point in the body to support and nourish the head, face, and brain. All of the yang channels also meet in the head. The head is thus considered the most yang part of the body and the meeting point of yang. The yang qi nourishes the five senses and the multitude of physiological functions. Failure of the yang activity may result in a broad condition of neurological and psychological malfunction.

After the clear yang has been processed in the head it is automatically transformed into turbid qi, which is a mixture of spent yang and waste products from the brain's metabolic processes. The turbid qi has no remaining nourishing qualities; on the contrary, it can disturb and block the clear yang, and thus have a very negative influence on the normal activities of the brain and nervous system. It is therefore important that the turbid qi be discharged from the head. The turbid qi, as distinguished from the clear yang, is associated with yin and has an innate tendency to descend. Under normal circumstances there is a natural exchange between the turbid qi and the clear yang. This interaction maintains a clear environ-

Fig. 1   ment in the head, and a sharp and clear consciousness will result.

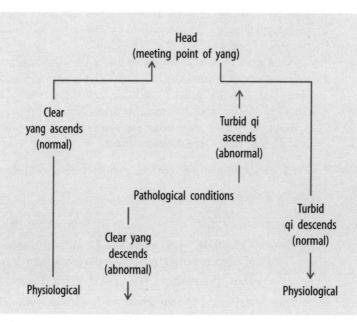

Cause of disease	Emotional pathogenic factor

One week ago after an emotional upset the symptoms became very severe. At the same time the patient developed distention in the intercostal and hypochondriac regions. This implies that an Organ is affected. Thus the cause of disease is internal.

Site of disease	Heart, Spleen, and Liver

The main evidence suggesting a Heart disorder is the palpitations and dream-disturbed sleep.

The main evidence suggesting a Spleen disturbance is the poor appetite, lassitude, and epigastric and abdominal distention.

Evidence of a Liver disorder is the wiry pulse and distention in the intercostal and hypochondriac region.

Pathological change

As stated earlier, the exchange between the clear yang and turbid yin is an essential foundation for good health. Two different factors can cause the failure of the clear yang to ascend, both of which are common in the clinic. The first is due to deficiency of clear yang which is simply not strong enough to reach the head, and the second to obstruction of the clear yang by pathological products, including phlegm, congested fluids, and stagnated blood. This patient's symptoms suggest the first category.

The history and symptoms in this case reveal a pattern of irregular dizziness. During the last week the symptoms worsened, accompanied by lassitude, poor appetite, and abdominal distention, exhibiting an obvious pattern of Spleen qi deficiency which prevented the ascension of Spleen qi.

The main function of the Spleen is to transform and transport food. The transformation process involves the breakdown of food into nutritive essence. The process of transportation dispatches the nutritive essence to the head and also to the Heart, Lung, and other parts of the body. This process is known as the raising of clear yang. Because the Spleen qi is deficient, the patient's appetite is poor and her abdomen is distended; her limbs and body have also become malnourished, resulting in general lassitude. Furthermore, the clear yang is not produced in sufficient quantity, the exchange relationship between the clear yang and the turbid yin is thrown out of balance, and hence the turbid yin cannot descend. This causes the dizziness and drowsiness. The activity of qi in the head is disturbed by the retention of turbid yin, and the obstruction causes occasional headaches.

Fig. 2

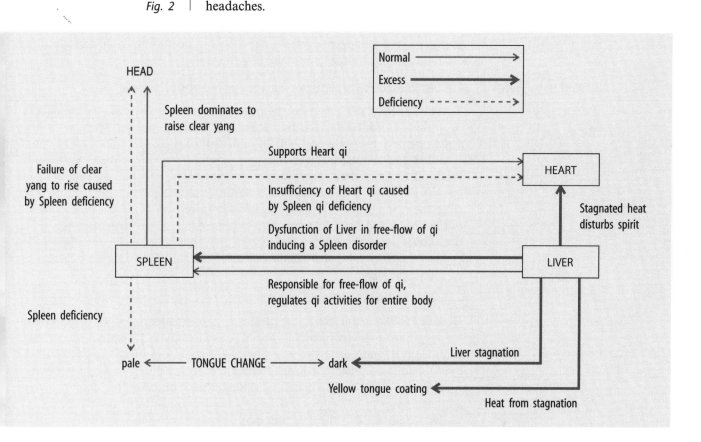

The emotional pathogenic factor has played a major role in the onset of this disorder. The Liver is commonly influenced by emotional upset. This can impair the free-flowing nature of the Liver. In this case there is distention in the hypochondriac and intercostal regions, a classic manifestation of stagnation of Liver qi. A problem in the Liver may sometimes induce a problem in the Spleen, or, if a Spleen disorder is already present, the Liver disorder can make the condition worse. This suggests a pattern of wood (Liver) invading earth (Spleen), as occurred in this case.

The bitter taste in the mouth and dry stools indicate heat in the body. This particular pattern of heat is caused by the stagnation of qi, and is called *yù rè* in Chinese. The qi is associated with yang. When the qi is obstructed for an extended period of time its accumulation will tend to develop into heat, and thus the yang nature of the qi will assert itself. In this case it was clearly caused by an emotional pathogenic factor. The stagnation of Liver qi led to the development of internal heat, and there has been some consumption of the fluids, as indicated by the dry stools. But if the heat were strong, i.e., Liver fire, the patient would be thirsty. There is no complaint of thirst in this case, thus the body fluids have not been severely consumed.

Heat disturbs the spirit and leads to palpitations and dream-disturbed sleep. The deficiency of the Spleen has led to deficiency of qi, and then to poor circulation; this was further affected by the stagnation of Liver qi. These factors explain why the tongue is pale and dark. The patient has heat from stagnation, thus the tongue coating is a little yellow and the pulse is rapid.

Pattern of disease

This is an interior pattern of disease, the evidence for which includes the emotional upset and the deficiency of Spleen qi.

There is also a pattern of heat. The main evidence for this is the dream-disturbed sleep, palpitations, yellow tongue coating, and the slippery and rapid pulse.

In this case there is a combination of deficiency and excessive patterns. The lassitude and poor appetite indicate deficiency, while the intercostal and hypochondriac distention indicate a pattern of excess.

Additional notes

1. Is there deficiency of Heart qi, yin, or blood in this case?

There is Heart qi deficiency, as the deficiency in the Spleen reduces the quantity of qi that is produced. This may affect the Heart qi and the spirit, and hence symptoms like lassitude and palpitations may emerge.

When there is deficiency of Heart yin or blood, malnourishment of the spirit, head and eyes may occur. Symptoms such as insomnia, palpitations, blurred vision, and dizziness may be present. In addition there may be general symptoms of blood deficiency such as pallor of the face, lips, finger nails, and tongue, and numbness of the hands and feet. Or there may be symptoms of yin deficiency like malar flush, burning in the five centers, etc. In this case, besides the dream-disturbed sleep and pale tongue, there is no evidence to support a diagnosis of Heart yin or blood deficiency.

2. Is there a preponderance of Liver yang or Liver fire ascending?

Dizziness is frequently seen in the patterns of a preponderance of Liver yang (internal wind) or Liver fire rising up. The cause of this patient's disease was an emotional upset; moreover there is obvious discomfort in the intercostal and hypochondriac regions. Both of these symptoms are also commonly seen when Liver fire or Liver yang ascends, and it is important to correctly differentiate these patterns.

Dizziness can be caused by internal wind or fire. Sometimes the two pathogenic factors combine in which case the dizziness is caused by wind-fire. It is usually very severe, and the accompanying symptoms reflect a general picture of hyperactivity including restlessness, tinnitus, insomnia, and irritability.

This patient has symptoms of diminished function, such as the drowsiness and general lassitude, and therefore is only suffering from stagnation of Liver qi. There is no preponderance of Liver yang. Furthermore, the true cause of the dizziness is deficiency brought on by the inability of the depleted clear yang to nourish the head.

3. What is the cause of the greasy, thick tongue coating and the slippery pulse in this case?

The deficiency of Spleen qi impairs its ability to metabolize water, and this encourages the formation of dampness. As previously mentioned, there is heat from stagnation, and this heat has combined with the dampness, thus the yin and yang pathogenic factors have united. This explains why the tongue coating is thick, yellow and greasy and the pulse is slippery and rapid. Compared with the main problem, however, the dampness is not obvious and is thus less important.

4. Is there any blood stasis?

In the section on pathological change we noted that the dark tongue body was said to reflect poor circulation of blood. If there are no other definite indications of blood stasis, then the tongue indicates just a *tendency* towards blood stasis. Because no other symptoms exist in this case, there is no blood stasis.

Conclusion

1. According to the eight principles:
   Interior, heat, deficient and excessive pattern.
2. According to etiology:
   Emotional pathogenic factor.
3. According to Organ theory:
   Spleen and Heart qi deficiency.
   Liver qi stagnation leading to heat.

Treatment principle

1. Reinforce the Heart and Spleen qi.
2. Regulate the Liver qi.
3. Clear the heat.

Selection of points

P-6 *(nei guan)*
Sp-4 *(gong sun)*
Liv-5 *(li gou)*
G-13 *(ben shen)*
G-44 *(zu qiao yin)*

Explanation of points

P-6 *(nei guan)* is selected to reinforce the Heart qi and calm the spirit. Like the Liver, it is associated with a terminal yin channel. This point can also help regulate the Liver qi.

Sp-4 *(gong sun)* regulates the Stomach and Spleen qi, and also regulates the function of the Large Intestine. In addition, it helps to remove dampness and phlegm.

The combination of these first two points regulates the qi of the upper and middle burners.

Liv-5 *(li gou)* is the connecting point of the Liver channel. It regulates Liver qi and removes stagnation.

G-13 *(ben shen)* clears heat, alleviates lateral headaches, and calms the spirit. All three functions of this point are well-indicated for this case.

G-44 *(zu qiao yin)* is an effective point for removing heat from the lesser yang, and also calms the spirit.

Combination of points

G-13 *(ben shen)* and G-44 *(zu qiao yin)* are both from the lesser yang channel, one at the lowest point of the body, the other at the highest. Both points clear heat from the Liver and Gallbladder and eliminate the dream-disturbed sleep caused by Liver or Gallbladder heat.

Follow-up

After two treatments spaced two days apart, the patient felt that her spirit was clearer, the episodes of dizziness had become less frequent, and the headache was gone. However, her sleep remained poor and she still complained of distention in the intercostal, hypochondriac, and epigastric regions. Treatment continued on alternate days for an additional week, after which she was symptom free and was discharged. She returned two months later with a complaint of abdominal distention, but had no relapse of dizziness.

CASE 10: **Female, age 44**

Main complaint

Dizziness

History

The patient has a history of dizziness for just one week. There was no obvious causative factor. She has nausea but no vomiting. She does not have any whirling or spinning sensation with the dizziness, but occasionally has mild tinnitus. She complains of a poor appetite and mild pain in the epigastric and abdominal regions. She does not like to drink water and avoids cold foods. Her urination and stool are normal.

Tongue

Pale and flabby body with small purple spots, thin tongue coating, middle and back is white and moist

Pulse

Slippery

Analysis of symptoms

1. Dizziness, tinnitus—clear yang cannot rise.
2. Nausea, poor appetite, abdominal pain—
   dysfunction of Spleen qi ascending and Stomach qi descending.
3. Pale, flabby tongue body, white moist coating—damp-cold.
4. Ecchymosis (purple spots) on tongue body—blood stasis.
5. Slippery pulse—retention of pathogenic dampness.

Basic theory of case

The concept of phlegm *(tán)* is very broad in Chinese medicine. It encompasses sputum from the respiratory tract, which is known as visible or formed phlegm. However, when only symptoms of phlegm are evident in certain Organs, channels, collaterals, and the subcutaneous tissues, it is known as invisible or formless phlegm.

Many patterns of disease in Chinese medicine involve phlegm, e.g., phlegm misting the Heart, which can result in the patient muttering to himself or behaving in an illogical manner. When the retention of phlegm is in the channels and collaterals, the patient can develop numbness or paresthesia on the limbs and body, or hemiplegia. When the phlegm is retained subcutaneously soft nodules may emerge. Most of these disorders are caused by invisible phlegm.

Invisible phlegm tends to accumulate in local areas, and this may be in the channels, vessels, or one or more of the Organs; in this case the normal function of the Organ or tissue will be disrupted by such accumulation. Thus the diagnosis of invisible phlegm can be made according to the symptoms and the pathological change.

Cause of disease

Phlegm

The dizziness here is accompanied by nausea and poor appetite. This confirms the presence of retained phlegm in the Organs, and a disruption in the directional flow of qi. The white, moist tongue coating and slippery pulse likewise confirm the presence of phlegm.

Site of disease

Head and Stomach

The dizziness and tinnitus indicate that the site of disease is the head.

The nausea, poor appetite, and abdominal pain form the principal evidence to suggest that the Stomach is involved.

Pathological change

In Chinese medicine a diagnosis of a phlegm pattern is based on the symptoms and pathological change, and whether the phlegm can be seen or not is of no significance. This patient has dizziness accompanied by nausea and other symptoms of middle burner disharmony. The basic pathological change involves the reversal of Stomach qi, which inhibits the ascending of clear yang. The disruption of the metabolism in the middle burner is a consequence of the retained phlegm.

Fig. 3

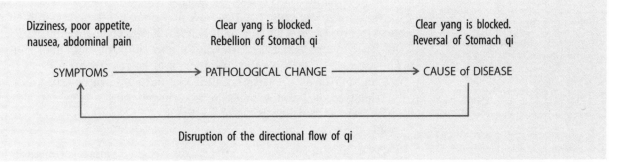

Disruption of the directional flow of qi

The retained phlegm in the middle burner blocks the ascension of clear yang and the turbid qi cannot descend from the head. This results in dizziness. The ear, which receives nourishment from the clear yang, is also affected. Tinnitus is caused by a preponderance of turbid qi in the head, and a failure of the clear yang to nourish the sensory organs.

Phlegm in the middle burner disrupts the directional flow of qi. Nausea is a common symptom of phlegm retention, and if the nausea is severe there may also be vomiting. The retention of phlegm in the Stomach causes the patient's poor appetite. There is no deficiency of body fluids in this case, thus the patient has no desire to drink.

Phlegm is a yin pathogenic factor which can block the yang qi. The yang qi of the middle burner is inhibited, resulting in epigastric and abdominal pain. Cold food can further weaken the yang qi, and the pain will then become worse. This explains why the patient cannot take cold foods. Bowel movement and urination are normal, thus the lower burner is unaffected.

The pale, flabby tongue, white, moist coating, and slippery pulse suggest retention of phlegm. The ecchymosis on the tongue body reflects blood stasis. There are two causes for this symptom: phlegm blocks the qi, which inhibits the circulation of blood; and cold constricts the flow of blood and eventually leads to stagnation. The blood stasis is not severe in this case.

Pattern of disease

The retention of phlegm in the middle burner indicates an interior pattern.

The presence of phlegm and absence of thirst indicate a cold pattern. This is confirmed by the pale tongue and white coating.

The pathogenic factors, i.e., phlegm and cold, are very strong; moreover, there is no weakness of antipathogenic factor, thus the patient has an excessive pattern of disease.

Additional notes

1. What is the cause of the phlegm?

Phlegm is a consequence of impaired water metabolism. Malfunction of the Lung, Spleen, or Kidney can give rise to phlegm.

In this case the phlegm is associated with a disorder of the Spleen and Stomach, and from the pale nature of the tongue we can surmise that the patient has a slight yang deficiency. The water metabolism is therefore weak, and the ensuing dampness can produce phlegm. The phlegm remains in the Stomach and Spleen where it further impairs the function of the middle burner. There is no evidence to suggest Lung or Kidney involvement in this case.

2. How does one differentiate the symptom of dizziness from other pathogenic factors?

In Chinese medicine there are many other causes of dizziness besides phlegm, e.g., Liver yang or fire rising, qi and blood deficiency, yin or vital essence deficiency, etc. The keys to differentiating dizziness are summarized at the end of this chapter.

In general, dizziness caused by phlegm tends to be severe. Some patients even develop a whirling sensation that may occasionally interfere with their ability to stand or even sit up. This type of dizziness will be accompanied by nausea or vomiting. The vomitus is like clear water, or it may be frothy and bubbly but still clear. This type of vomitus is called *xián*, or 'oral mucus'. In other cases the vomitus is thick and turbid. It is then called *tán*, meaning simply phlegm or sputum.

This type of dizziness tends to be recurrent, and attacks can last a few days or few weeks. However, between the bouts of disease there will be no symptoms at all.

3. Does this patient have a deficient or excessive pattern of disease?

When we analyzed the cause of the phlegm we referred to a history of yang deficiency in the middle burner, as well as the patient's poor appetite and pale, flabby tongue. Yang deficiency of the middle burner seems quite probable in this case. However, based on the other symptoms and the duration of the disorder, we know that retention of phlegm is the main problem. The poor appetite can be explained by the retention of phlegm, and the pale tongue can be caused by yang deficiency or phlegm-cold. At present the excessive phlegm pattern is more important since the indications of a deficient pattern in this patient are not obvious.

Conclusion

1. According to the eight principles:
   Interior, cold, and excessive pattern.

2. According to etiology:
   Retention of phlegm.

3. According to Organ theory:
   Retention of phlegm in the Stomach which inhibits the ascension of clear yang.

Treatment principle

Remove the phlegm and regulate the qi.

Selection of points

S-8 *(tou wei)*
G-20 *(feng chi)*
CV-12 *(zhong wan)*
S-25 *(tian shu)*
S-36 *(zu san li)* on one side
S-40 *(feng long)* on one side

Explanation of points

S-8 *(tou wei)* is on the Stomach channel. It is indicated to clear turbid qi from the head, and thus is a good point for yang brightness disorders with symptoms like dizziness or headache.

G-20 *(feng chi)* is called the 'wind pool' in Chinese. Dizziness is associated with wind in Chinese medicine, and G-20 *(feng chi)* has a strong effect in expelling both internal and external wind. The Gallbladder has an exterior-interior relationship with the Liver. This point regulates the qi of the lesser yang channel and is used to promote the free-flowing function of Liver qi that is helpful in removing phlegm.

CV-12 *(zhong wan)* is the alarm point of the Stomach. This point is very effective in harmonizing the middle burner. It also regulates the qi and removes obstruction from the middle burner. It will therefore help remove the phlegm and alleviate the epigastric pain.

S-25 *(tian shu)* is a good point for regulating the yang brightness channel, thus both the Stomach and Large Intestine are regulated by this point. It will therefore help relieve the abdominal pain and stagnation of qi in the middle burner.

S-36 *(zu san li)* and S-40 *(feng long)* help remove phlegm and promote the function of the middle burner.

Follow-up

This patient was treated only three times on alternate days, after which she had no dizziness or other symptoms. She was seen six months later in connection with an unrelated problem and reported that she had experienced no further dizziness.

CASE 11: **Male, age 35**

Main complaint

Dizziness

History

This patient has a history of episodic dizziness for the last two years, and around the same time was diagnosed with hypertension. His blood pressure is very unstable, and dizziness occurs each time the blood pressure rises. The dizziness has been relieved by Western medicine.

This young man was very hot-tempered and irritable. After each fit of anger the hypertension and dizziness became worse. The most recent onset began two weeks ago, and again the symptoms were caused by an outburst of anger, but this time the Western medicine did not relieve his dizziness. It is so severe that it affects his ability to walk. He sleeps fitfully and suffers from general lassitude. The patient's appetite is unaffected by his main complaint. He has a red complexion and red eyes.

Tongue

Red tongue body, thin and yellow coating

Pulse

Wiry and thin
Blood pressure: 170/90mmHg

Analysis of symptoms

1. Hot temper, irritability—malfunction of the Liver qi.
2. Dizziness—heat rising to disturb the head.
3. Unsound sleep—disturbance of the spirit.
4. General lassitude—qi disorder.
5. Red face and eyes, red tongue, yellow coating—heat pattern.
6. Wiry pulse—Liver disorder.

Basic theory of case

The Liver governs the free-flowing of qi, and this means that the qi of the entire body can be regulated by the Liver. The Liver continuously removes obstructions in the body to ensure the directional flow of yang qi. The Liver qi is very active and has an innate tendency to ascend. In Chinese medicine the Liver is called *yáng gāng zhī zàng,* or 'the yin Organ of yang and rigidity.' This explains why both the Liver qi and yang have a tendency towards excess. The Liver yin and blood are thus vulnerable since they may often be attacked and consumed by Liver yang. This is why the Liver yin and blood are always involved when there is deficiency. Thus a Liver disorder typically exhibits an excess of Liver yang and deficiency of Liver yin.

Fig. 4

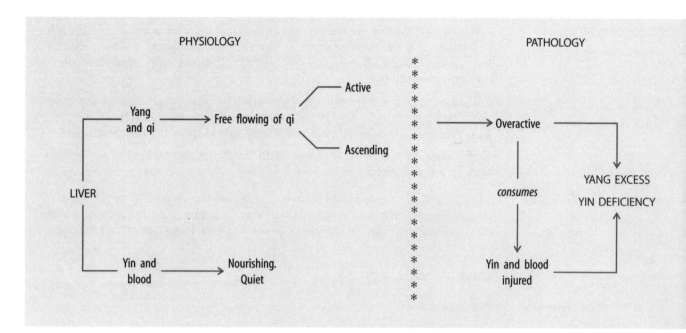

The terms Liver yang rising or preponderance of Liver yang refer to a hyperfunction of the Liver yang in ascending. Emotional pathogenic factors can cause this disorder, especially sudden and strong anger. This type of emotional outburst has a malevolent influence on the qi, which causes heat from stagnation. When there is both stagnant qi and heat the Liver yin will be slightly consumed. This is called stagnant Liver heat. At this stage the condition is still excessive in nature.

The Liver and Kidney are both in the lower burner and share the same source of yin. Long-term deficiency of Liver yin can injure the Kidney yin, and the balance between the yin and yang aspects will thereby be disrupted. The manifestations of this pattern will appear to be excessive, but the root of the disorder is one of deficiency. This pattern is commonly known as preponderance of Liver yang.

Fig. 5

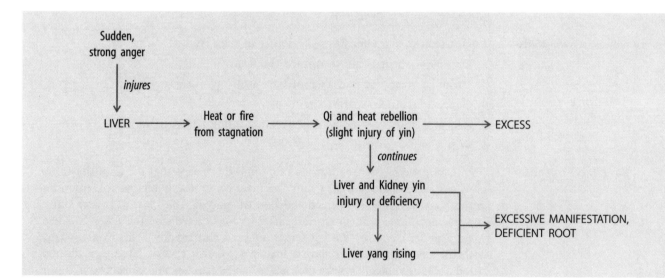

Cause of disease	Emotional pathogenic factor

This patient has a hot, quick temper and is frequently irritable. Each onset of symptoms is caused by a strong emotional outburst. That means there is a concrete link between his emotional state and his disease.

Site of disease	Head and Liver

The patient has obvious dizziness to the extent that his ability to walk is affected. This indicates that the head is disturbed.

The irritability, hot temper, and wiry pulse indicate a Liver disorder.

Pathological change	

The patient is frequently irritable and has a hot temper, thus there is a continual imbalance in the yin and yang aspects of the Liver. There are two possible causes for this imbalance: the preponderance of yang may be congenital, or it may be linked to a recurrent form of emotional pathogenic factor. This develops during childhood and adolescence and leaves the person with a volatile tendency to develop heat from stagnation. As mentioned earlier, this gives rise to a pattern of yang excess and insufficiency of yin.

The heat from stagnation is a yang pathogenic factor which rises up to disturb the head, affecting the qi and blood in the channels and collaterals, and causing dizziness. This will often cause a heavy sensation in the head and light feeling in the feet, as if one were walking on cotton wool. An unusual type of 'whole-head headache' may also occur.

The sudden outbursts of emotion are destructive of the free-flowing action of the Liver qi, thus each outburst of anger causes a recurrence of his main symptoms. The blood will follow the qi, and as the Liver qi over-ascends, the flow of blood will reverse upwards; thus the complexion and eyes become red. In severe cases sudden hemorrhage in the upper aspect of the body may occur, e.g., spontaneous nosebleeds or even vomiting of blood.

The Heart is the house of the spirit. When heat rises upwards it disturbs the spirit, which explains why the patient complains of poor sleep.

The patient has a two-year history of dizziness. His main symptoms indicate heat and excess caused by the stagnation of Liver qi. There is also injury to the Liver yin aspect, the main indication being the thin pulse. If the pulse were typically wiry it would indicate impairment of the Liver's main (yang) function, but the thin pulse suggests an injury to the yin aspect. His general condition does not exhibit any significant yin-deficient symptoms, hence it is not severe.

General lassitude reflects an injury to the qi, for which there are two possible causes. The Liver disorder first affects the free-flowing of qi, and then the Spleen's ability to transport and transform. This is known as wood (Liver) invading earth (Spleen). Second, the heat from stagnation over-ascends and consumes the qi, causing lassitude. In this case the second hypothesis is more likely.

Fig. 6

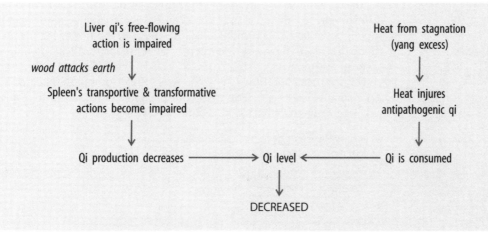

The red tongue and yellow coating clearly indicate the presence of heat. The wiry and thin pulse was previously explained.

Pattern of disease

The emotional pathogenic factor has attacked the Liver directly, thus the patient has an interior pattern.

The patient is hot tempered with a red complexion and red eyes. The tongue is red with a yellow coating. There is thus a pattern of heat.

Because the case is characterized by excessive heat, it is also a pattern of excess.

Additional notes

1. Is there a pattern of deficiency in this case?

There are two symptoms that possibly indicate a pattern of deficiency. A thin pulse generally indicates deficiency of qi and blood or yin. Another possible cause is retention of dampness. In this case the only possible reason is an injury to the yin. However, there is no other evidence to support this except the pulse. The injury to the yin is therefore very mild.

General lassitude is usually associated with a pattern of deficiency. However, in this case the lassitude is part of an injury to the qi which was caused by the excessive heat. The symptoms and pathological change are different from those of Spleen qi deficiency, thus a diagnosis of Spleen qi deficiency is unsupported.

2. What are the keys to distinguishing the three types of Liver yang disorder?

The three types of Liver yang disorder are stagnant Liver heat, Liver fire rising, and preponderance of Liver yang. Stagnant heat and Liver fire rising both are hot and excessive in nature, but the heat from stagnation is not as severe as Liver fire rising. There are other important differences in symptoms as well. Heat from stagnation tends to show an acute pattern of emotional depressive behavior that accompanies the heat symptoms, while Liver fire rising has stronger heat symptoms that cause obvious manifestations of consumption of the body fluids; the depressive symptoms are always milder in this pattern, however. In the clinic some practitioners draw no distinction between these two patterns, but the treatment principle and point selection should be adjusted according to the differentiation.

Preponderance of Liver yang is regarded as a combination of excess and deficiency patterns. There are two main causes for this pattern. Heat from stagnation or Liver fire may consume the Liver yin and cause yin deficiency, or the deficiency of Liver yin may also be caused by a chronic disease or by old age. The symptoms of this pattern can be divided into two groups, one of which reflects a preponderance of yang, and the other deficient yin.

The preponderance of yang can easily be mistaken for a pattern of Liver fire because the symptoms of both are very similar, but the pattern of Liver fire rising will always exhibit symptoms of more severe heat with consumption of the body fluids. There will also be very pronounced insomnia, severe restlessness, a hot sensation over the entire body, and great thirst.

In the clinic it is important to distinguish between these patterns. They have different causes, manifestations, and pathological change, and the point selection should be adjusted accordingly. Heat from stagnation or Liver fire are both excessive patterns that require treatment that removes the heat. Points that regulate Liver qi and remove qi stagnation are used for the former; points that clear heat or fire are used for the latter. The root of the preponderance of Liver yang is deficiency of Liver yin. The treatment principle is primarily to nourish the Liver yin, and only secondarily to sedate the Liver yang.

Conclusion

1. According to the eight principles:
   Interior, heat, excessive.

2. According to etiology:
   Emotional pathogenic factor.

3. According to Organ theory:
   Heat from stagnation in the Liver.

Treatment principle | Regulate the Liver qi, clear the heat, and calm the spirit.

Selection of points

G-13 *(ben shen)*
G-20 *(feng chi)*
LI-11 *(qu chi)* through to H-3 *(shao hai)*
G-34 *(yang ling quan)*
Liv-2 *(xing jian)*

Explanation of points

G-13 *(ben shen)* clears heat and calms the spirit. The poor sleep and dizziness make this point most suitable.

G-20 *(feng chi)* is the meeting point of the yang linking vessel and lesser yang channels. It helps clear the heat via the yang linking vessel aspect. Moreover, from the lesser yang aspect the point can be used to resolve wind (both internal and external), which is helpful in regulating the Liver qi.

LI-11 *(qu chi)* through to H-3 *(shao hai)*: Both of these points are sea points and are effective in clearing heat. One point is from the yang brightness and the other from the lesser yin. The sea point on the yang brightness channel is particularly good for removing heat, as the yang brightness is rich in qi and blood. This point promotes the drawing of heat from the lesser yang. H-3 *(shao hai)* calms the spirit and clears heat from the lesser yin.

G-34 *(yang ling quan)* is the sea point of the lesser yang. It helps remove the heat from the lesser yang and terminal yin channels, and also regulates the qi of these two channels.

Liv-2 *(xing jian)* is a spring point and is effective in removing heat from the qi level. The use of G-34 *(yang ling quan)* and Liv-2 *(xing jian)* is well indicated when there is heat in either the Gallbladder or Liver.

Follow-up

After the first treatment the patient felt much improved. He experienced less dizziness, and his blood pressure dropped to 150/90mmHg. The next day all of his symptoms returned, however, and his blood pressure again rose to 160/100mmHg. He was treated three times a week for a total of fifteen treatments. The intervals between dizzy spells became longer and longer during this time, and his blood pressure stabilized. However, he still complained of irritability, his tongue remained red, and his pulse was still wiry and thin.

The treatment principle was therefore changed to regulating the Liver qi, clearing the Liver heat, and calming the spirit. The new point prescription was as follows:

P-6 *(nei guan)*
CV-17 *(shan zhong)*
G-34 *(yang ling quan)*
Liv-2 *(xing jian)*
G-13 *(ben shen)*
GV-24 *(shen ting)*

After two more weeks of treatment he became much less irritable and was discharged. His blood pressure stabilized at 150/90mmHg during a six month follow-up period.

CASE 12: **Male, age 57**

Main complaint | Dizziness

History

Nine years ago the patient developed very severe dizziness. He experienced a whirling sensation as if he were on a small boat in rough seas. Sometimes the onset was so severe that he could hardly walk. The accompanying symptoms were vomiting, high-frequency tinnitus, and low blood pressure. He has had two relapses of a similar pattern over the past nine years.

Two months ago the dizziness recurred, and the patient found that whenever he read, the dizziness became worse. His balance was very poor, his appetite diminished, and there was nausea and a tendency to vomit. There was an abnormal sensation in the abdominal and epigastric regions. He expectorated small quantities of phlegm. The patient has also noticed that his weight has decreased, he belches a lot, and frequently passes gas. Bowel movements are normal, but his rectum is slightly prolapsed. The patient has slight urinary frequency. Over the past few days he developed urticaria around the entire body, accompanied by pruritus, which makes it very difficult to sleep. He also has nightmares.

Tongue	Pale body, white and thin coating
Pulse	Wiry, thin, forceless
Analysis of symptoms	1. Dizziness, tinnitus, whirling sensation—clear yang cannot ascend.
	2. Nausea, vomiting, belching—reversal of Stomach qi.
	3. Poor appetite, reduced body weight, prolapse of rectum— Spleen qi deficiency.
	4. Urticaria, pruritus of the skin— invasion of superficial tissues by pathogenic wind.
	5. Thin, forceless pulse, pale tongue—deficient disorder.

Basic theory of case

The Spleen governs the ascending action of qi, which is part of the Spleen's function of transformation and transportation. The Spleen dispatches the food essence to the upper burner and the Lungs, and then disperses it throughout the body, as described in case number 9. The Spleen's ascending action includes its ability to hold the Organs in place, particularly the Stomach, Spleen, Liver, Kidneys, uterus, and Intestines.

Each of the Organs has a yin and a yang aspect. The yang aspect controls the functional activity and the yin aspect governs the substance of the Organ itself. Although the yang qi of each Organ is specialized, all yang qi shares the characteristic of raising the Organs upward to hold them in their proper positions. The strength of the yang qi in holding up an Organ is dependent upon the weight of that Organ; thus the maintenance of normal position of an Organ is dependent upon the health of the yang qi.

The Spleen continuously replenishes the yang qi 'holding' aspect of the Organs and is thus primarily responsible for the holding function. The Spleen's failure to nourish and support the other Organs eventually impairs their ability to hold in place, and it is then that an Organ can prolapse. In Chinese medicine this is called 'sinking of the Spleen qi'. *See Fig. 7.*

Cause of disease

Phlegm

The dizziness accompanied by nausea and poor appetite confirms the presence of phlegm, which upsets the directional flow of qi.

Site of disease

Head, Stomach, and Spleen

The dizziness and tinnitus suggest involvement of the head.
The nausea, vomiting, and belching indicate a Stomach disorder.
The poor appetite, emaciation, and prolapsed rectum indicate a Spleen disorder.

Pathological change

Although there are many causes of dizziness, phlegm is the most common. There is a Chinese saying, "No phlegm, no dizziness." Phlegm blocks the normal

Fig. 7

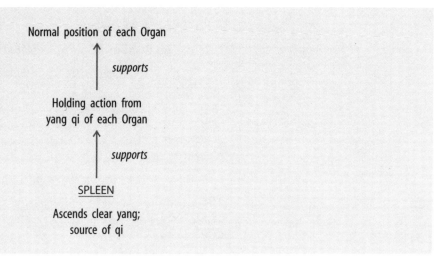

Normal position of each Organ

↑

supports

Holding action from
yang qi of each Organ

↑

supports

SPLEEN

Ascends clear yang;
source of qi

ascension of clear yang and causes dizziness. However, it should be noted that phlegm is not the only cause of dizziness. For example, in case number 9 it was the deficiency of Spleen qi that led to dizziness, as the clear yang was simply too weak to ascend. By contrast, case number 10 displayed a typical pattern of retained phlegm leading to dizziness.

This case is a combination of Spleen deficiency and retention of phlegm, which is also very common in the clinic. Because the phlegm obstructs the circulation of qi, the clear yang cannot rise to support the head, face, ears, and eyes. Thus the patient experiences dizziness, tinnitus, and a whirling sensation. The phlegm that is retained in the Stomach can cause reversal of the Stomach qi, the symptoms of which are nausea with a tendency to vomit.

Because the Spleen qi is deficient, its transportive and transformative functions are impaired, which in turn reduces the patient's appetite. The Spleen governs the muscles, and the shortage of food essence causes malnourishment of the muscles. The lack of nourishment will gradually cause loss of body weight.

At the same time, the deficiency of Spleen qi can aggravate the failure of the clear yang to rise. Everyone knows that physical activity consumes the body's energy, but mental activity involving a lot of thinking also consumes the body's qi. This may explain the deterioration in the patient's symptoms occasioned by reading.

The deficiency of Spleen qi weakens its holding action, which in this case has led to the prolapse of the rectum, the most common symptom of Spleen qi sinking. The weakness of the Spleen and the presence of phlegm prevents the qi from rising, thus the qi remains in the Large Intestine and causes flatulence.

Urticaria in Chinese medicine is called wind rash *(fēng zhěn)*. This is caused by invasion of the body surface by pathogenic wind, which obstructs the skin, interstices, and pores.

The pale tongue and thin, forceless pulse are symptoms of deficiency.

Pattern of disease

This patient has both an interior and an exterior pattern. The interior pattern is suggested by the retention of phlegm which prevents the qi from rising. The exterior skin pattern is caused by invasion of the body surface by wind.

There are no heat symptoms in this case. The pulse and tongue have cold characteristics, suggesting a pattern of cold.

There is a combination of excess and deficiency. The excessive pattern is indicated by the presence of phlegm and includes the symptoms of dizziness, nausea, and vomiting. The deficiency pattern is evidenced by the hypofunction of the Spleen in transforming and transporting, manifested in the poor appetite, weight loss, and prolapsed rectum.

Additional notes

1. Is the production of phlegm related to the deficiency of the Spleen?

The Spleen is responsible for water metabolism. When the Spleen is deficient there may be retention of congested fluids or dampness, a possible source of phlegm. From another viewpoint the phlegm can be seen as an independent pathogenic factor. Retention of phlegm can restrain the Spleen qi, eventually leading to Spleen qi deficiency. These two causes frequently affect one another. In this case the phlegm is caused by Spleen qi deficiency.

2. Is there a relationship between the interior and exterior patterns?

The urticaria is caused by an invasion of pathogenic wind and its history in this case is very short, yet the dizziness has a two-month history. The dizziness and urticaria can therefore be regarded as separate problems.

3. What is the cause of the urinary frequency?

There are commonly two causes of this problem. The first is damp-heat. In addition to the frequent urination, the patient may experience a sensation of heat, urgency, and pain when urine is being passed. The urine will be yellow. The second possible cause of this problem is qi deficiency. The Bladder is unable to control itself, leading to frequent urination. Because, as we have seen, this patient has a deficiency of qi, his condition thus corresponds to the second pattern.

In the clinic we know that severe hypofunction of the Bladder is caused by Kidney qi deficiency, but the frequency of urination must be very marked to make that diagnosis. In this case the symptom of urinary frequency is accompanied by Spleen qi deficiency and is not especially severe, thus a diagnosis of Kidney qi deficiency is unwarranted.

4. What is the cause of the patient's insomnia?

The patient complains that the pruritus is affecting his sleep. This pattern is similar to the way in which pain disturbs sleep. It is therefore secondary insomnia and can only be relieved by treating the primary problem.

Still, this patient also has nightmares, so there must be some substantial internal cause, probably due to deficiency of the Heart and Gallbladder qi. Because the Spleen is very weak and there is retention of phlegm, as the source of qi the Spleen's deficiency can affect both of these Organs, and the presence of phlegm can impair the function of the Gallbladder. This is merely speculation, however. There are no other symptoms that would support this diagnosis. In particular, the patient does not frighten easily or have a timid personality. We therefore cannot make a concrete diagnosis. Only by carefully monitoring the patient's response to treatment can this diagnosis be tested.

5. Does the patient have a Liver disorder?

The patient has dizziness, insomnia, tinnitus, dream-disturbed sleep, and a wiry pulse. From this group of symptoms it is easy to diagnose a preponderance of Liver yang. However, Liver yang rising is a heat pattern, and here there are no manifestations of heat. The patient does not have a red complexion or red eyes, nor does he complain of irritability; in fact, he displays a pattern of cold. Retention of phlegm (present here) sometimes causes a wiry pulse, thus the pulse is quite understandable. However, it must be kept in mind that a weak Spleen could easily be attacked by an overactive Liver, thus the wiry pulse could be a warning sign of wood (Liver) invading earth (Spleen) in the near future.

Conclusion

1. According to the eight principles:
Both exterior and interior; cold; both excess and deficiency.
2. According to etiology:
Retention of phlegm.
Invasion of the superficial tissues by pathogenic wind, resulting in urticaria.
3. According to Organ theory:
Retention of phlegm in the middle burner leading to failure of the Spleen qi to ascend.
Spleen qi deficiency.

Treatment principle

1. Remove the phlegm.
2. Reinforce the Spleen qi and promote the clear yang.
3. Expel the pathogenic wind and relieve the urticaria.

Selection of points

CV-12 *(zhong wan)*
CV-14 *(ju que)*
GV-20 *(bai hui)*
G-20 *(feng chi)*
S-40 *(feng long)* through to B-58 *(fei yang)*

Explanation of points

CV-12 *(zhong wan)* is chosen for treating the Spleen qi deficiency and retention of phlegm in the middle burner. The two aspects of this point are contradictory in that one reduces while the other reinforces. Even manipulation of the needle should be used in this case. This is also the alarm point of the Stomach, which makes it a good choice for directing the rebellious Stomach qi downward.

CV-14 *(ju que)* helps remove obstruction and promotes the function of the Heart. It encourages the clear yang to rise. This point calms the spirit, supports the Heart qi, and relieves nightmares.

GV-20 *(bai hui)* regulates the yang of the body, thereby supporting the ascending action of the clear yang. It will also calm the spirit in this patient.

G-20 *(feng chi)* is a good point for arresting dizziness and clearing the spirit, as it regulates the qi activity of the head.

S-40 *(feng long)* is chosen to remove phlegm. It is the connecting point of the foot yang brightness and will thus affect both the Stomach and Spleen. The needle is threaded to B-58 *(fei yang)*, the connecting point of the foot greater yang. The greater yang governs the superficial tissues. By promoting the functions of the Organs and the superficial tissues, the pathogenic factors can be expelled from the surface of the skin.

Follow-up

The patient was treated twice a week for two weeks. At the end of the first week the skin rash and vertigo had disappeared, and during the second week he no longer complained of nausea. His appetite had also improved. The rectal prolapse remained as before, however, and the treatment principle was therefore changed to tonifying the Spleen and regulating the qi of the yin Organs. The following points were used:

B-13 *(fei shu)*
B-18 *(gan shu)*
B-20 *(pi shu)*
B-21 *(wei shu)*
GV-1 *(chang qiang)*

After two more weeks of treatment the rectal prolapse had improved.

Diagnostic principles for dizziness

In clinical practice dizziness is one of the most common complaints, ranging from a mild feeling of lightheadedness which does not interfere with normal activities, to severe vertigo with a whirling sensation that affects a person's balance such that he or she may even be afraid to open the eyes. This sensation is accompanied by severe nausea and vomiting.

Dizziness may present as an isolated symptom or be accompanied by headache. We are mainly concerned here with dizziness as the main complaint.

1. Classification and pathology of dizziness

In Chinese medicine the head is the meeting place of the yang channels and the governing vessel. A clear, calm spirit is one of the most important foundations of good health, and this is dependent on the upward-rising of clear yang. This process, in turn, is governed by the balance between yin and yang, and qi and blood. When these relationships are disturbed, the clear yang does not ascend and the patient becomes dizzy. Dizziness is classified on the basis of etiology.

Fig. 8

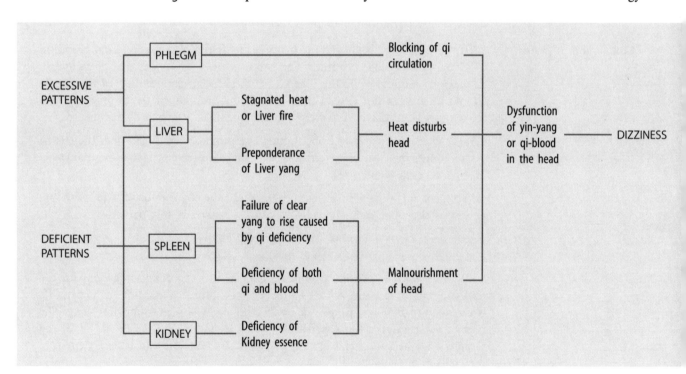

2. Key points in the diagnosis of dizziness

i. Retention of phlegm in the middle burner

Phlegm is a yin and substantial pathogenic factor which injures the yang qi of the body and also blocks the circulation of qi. When phlegm accumulates in the middle burner, the normal flow of qi in the Spleen and Stomach is impaired, the clear yang cannot ascend, and the turbid yin cannot descend.

The patient will complain of dizziness accompanied by nausea and vomiting. The dizziness may be mild or severe, and in the more serious case the patient will have a sensation of vertigo and may be unable to stand. The nausea and vomiting can be very severe because the pathogenic factor remains in the middle burner. *Tán yǐn* in Chinese means 'phlegm and congested fluids'. This term describes the type of vomitus produced in such cases, usually a yellowish, clear liquid rather than food. There may also be a stifling sensation in the chest, a heavy sensation around the body and limbs, anorexia, a greasy tongue coating, and a slippery pulse. These symptoms are characteristic of stagnant qi and excessive retention of phlegm.

ii. Liver disorders

There are three types of dizziness associated with disorders of the Liver: heat as a result of stagnant Liver qi, Liver fire rising, and preponderance of Liver yang.

The Liver stores the blood and governs the free-flowing of qi. Under normal circumstances the qi of the Liver tends to flow in an upward direction. If there is an imbalance between the Liver yin and yang, and the Liver qi thus rises too quickly and excessively to the head, the circulation of qi and blood in the head will be impaired and the patient will have headache, or headache and dizziness together. The dizziness can vary from mild to very severe, and is readily influenced by external stimuli such as emotional stress or noise. If the dizziness is severe, one may lose his balance when walking, but nausea, vomiting, and vertigo are rarely present. In most cases the patient will be irritable with a red face, tinnitus, a red tongue, and a rapid, wiry pulse indicating a preponderance of Liver yang or Liver qi disorder.

The distinguishing characteristics among these three disorders are as follows: Heat from stagnant Liver qi and Liver fire rising are patterns of excess, but the symptoms of Liver fire rising are more severe. The patient will usually present with severe insomnia, possibly with sleepless nights. He will also be very thirsty and have yellow urine, constipation, a red tongue with a thick yellow coating, and a wiry, rapid, and forceful pulse. These symptoms indicate very severe, excessive internal heat. While heat from stagnant Liver qi is also a pattern of internal heat, the symptoms are all milder.

Preponderance of Liver yang is a combination of excess and deficiency. This is a typical example of *běn xū biāo shí* or 'deficient root and excessive manifestation.' The patient with this pattern usually complains mainly of dizziness accompanied by anxiety, restlessness, insomnia, poor memory, weakness and soreness of the knee joints and lower back, a red tongue with a thin yellow coating, and a wiry, rapid, and thin pulse. The symptoms of yang preponderance mainly appear on the upper part of the body, and the yin deficiency symptoms on the lower part. This pattern is known as 'excess above, deficiency below'. This is heat from deficiency, thus the body fluids are rarely injured and the patient is unlikely to complain of thirst or a preference for cold beverages.

iii. Spleen deficiency and Kidney deficiency

The Spleen is the source of qi and blood and has the function of inducing the clear yang to rise. The Kidney stores the vital essence. Qi, blood, and vital essence are the substances which nourish the Organs, thus if the head is deprived of the nourishment and support of qi, blood, yin and yang because of Spleen or Kidney deficiency, the patient will experience dizziness. It will not be severe, but the condition is very chronic.

Dizziness caused by Spleen deficiency mainly involves the inability of the clear yang to ascend. Some patients will tell you that the dizziness is worse early in the morning when they wake, but improves or disappears when they get up and move about. This type of dizziness may be accompanied by general lassitude or fatigue, poor appetite, indigestion, a pale tongue, and a forceless pulse. The main distinction between Spleen qi deficiency and qi and blood deficiency is the absence of symptoms associated with blood deficiency, e.g., palpitations, facial pallor, or malnourishment of the nails.

The vital essence of the Kidney is the principal substance that nourishes the brain and spinal cord. When there is deficiency of vital essence, it is said that the 'sea of marrow loses nourishment.' The patient will experience dizziness with a light-headed sensation, accompanied by severe fatigue, poor concentration and impaired memory, and general symptoms such as soreness and weakness of the lower back and knee joints, nocturnal emissions with dreams, diminished tongue body with a very thin coating, and a thin, forceless pulse.

The entire diagnostic procedure for dizziness is summarized in the following chart.

Fig. 9

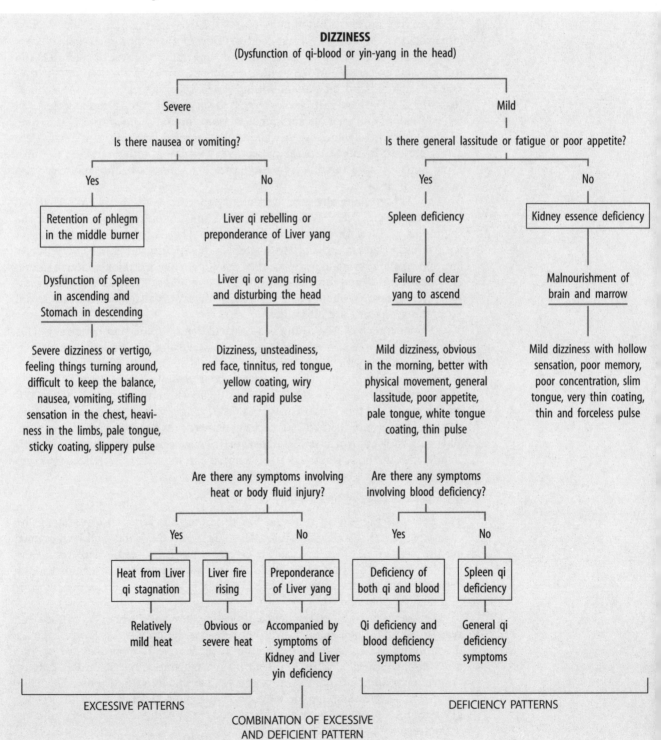

DIZZINESS
(Dysfunction of qi-blood or yin-yang in the head)

Severe — Is there nausea or vomiting?

Mild — Is there general lassitude or fatigue or poor appetite?

Severe: Yes / No
Mild: Yes / No

Yes (Severe)
Retention of phlegm in the middle burner

Dysfunction of Spleen in ascending and Stomach in descending

Severe dizziness or vertigo, feeling things turning around, difficult to keep the balance, nausea, vomiting, stifling sensation in the chest, heaviness in the limbs, pale tongue, sticky coating, slippery pulse

No (Severe)
Liver qi rebelling or preponderance of Liver yang

Liver qi or yang rising and disturbing the head

Dizziness, unsteadiness, red face, tinnitus, red tongue, yellow coating, wiry and rapid pulse

Are there any symptoms involving heat or body fluid injury?

Yes / No

Yes:
Heat from Liver qi stagnation — Relatively mild heat

Liver fire rising — Obvious or severe heat

No:
Preponderance of Liver yang — Accompanied by symptoms of Kidney and Liver yin deficiency

Yes (Mild)
Spleen deficiency

Failure of clear yang to ascend

Mild dizziness, obvious in the morning, better with physical movement, general lassitude, poor appetite, pale tongue, white tongue coating, thin pulse

Are there any symptoms involving blood deficiency?

Yes / No

Yes:
Deficiency of both qi and blood — Qi deficiency and blood deficiency symptoms

No:
Spleen qi deficiency — General qi deficiency symptoms

No (Mild)
Kidney essence deficiency

Malnourishment of brain and marrow

Mild dizziness with hollow sensation, poor memory, poor concentration, slim tongue, very thin coating, thin and forceless pulse

EXCESSIVE PATTERNS   DEFICIENCY PATTERNS

COMBINATION OF EXCESSIVE AND DEFICIENT PATTERN

Headache

CASE 13: **Female, age 52**

Main complaint

One-sided headache

History

The patient has a two year history of episodic, one-sided temporal headaches with no obvious precipitating cause. Three days ago she developed a right-sided headache following a family bereavement. The headache is fixed in the right temporal region and the pain becomes worse in spasms, especially when she feels particularly sad or upset. The pain interferes with sleep.

Her throat is dry and she feels thirsty and likes to drink. Her appetite is good but when she eats sweet things she has a feeling of distention in the epigastric region. She feels hot around the body and sweats easily. She has occasional chest pain, primarily on the left, but this is not severe. Her right upper arm feels uncomfortable, but there is no actual pain or limitation of movement.

Tongue

Dark red body with a yellow, slightly thick, greasy, and rather dry coating

Pulse

Sunken and wiry

Analysis of symptoms

1. Right-sided headache—obstruction in the channel.
2. Association of the pain with emotional change—lesser yang dysfunction.
3. Left-sided chest pain—poor circulation of qi in the chest.
4. Dry throat, general hot feeling, and thirst with a desire to drink—heat.
5. Red tongue with a dry, yellow coating—heat.
6. Sunken, wiry pulse—qi dysfunction.

Basic theory of case

There are two lesser yang channels, one involving the hand and one the foot, which pass between the greater yang and yang brightness channels on the limbs. In addition, the foot lesser yang channel runs along the lateral side of the body. In other words, the two channels run between the front and back, or the yin and yang aspects of the body.

The lesser yang channels are related to the Gallbladder and the Triple Burner. The Gallbladder and Liver have an exterior-interior relationship, which means that these two Organs have related functions. They both assist the free-flowing of qi, in particular by focusing on the direction of flow of the qi. This function also extends to the channels. In the *Inner Classic* this is known as the *shǎo yáng wéi shū*. This means 'lesser yang hinge' as it controls the flow of qi between yin and yang.

Qi regulates all the functions and relationships among qi, blood, and body fluids; the yin and yang Organs; and the channels and collaterals. In the Lungs, e.g., there is the dispersing and descending of qi wherein the Spleen and Stomach are responsible for raising the clear yang and causing the turbid yin to descend. There is also the relationship between the Heart and Kidney, in other words, the harmony between water and fire. All these functions involve qi activity; the Liver, Gallbladder, and lesser yang channels thus play a very important part in these physiological processes.

Cause of disease

Emotional change

This patient has no idea why her symptoms began two years ago, but the most recent episode is clearly related to emotional stress, and the pain becomes worse when she feels upset. Emotional change is therefore the main cause in this case.

Site of disease

Lesser yang channel and Gallbladder

This patient has a fixed, one-sided headache but no obvious problem with the yin Organs; it is therefore mainly the channel which is affected.

Emotional change aggravates the pain; the main Organ involved is therefore the Gallbladder.

Pathological change

The lesser yang controls qi activity; when there is a dysfunction, the qi may stagnate or even reverse its direction of flow. Emotional change can quickly influence the qi activity. In this case, the free-flowing of qi in the Gallbladder has become disrupted. There is qi stagnation in its related lesser yang channel. The lesser yang channel is located on the side of the head and behind the ear, and this is the main site of pain. The pain is episodic rather than continuous, which is a typical sign of qi stagnation. The pain in the right arm indicates that there is also some stagnation in the hand lesser yang channel.

Qi pertains to yang which is characterized by heat, thus qi stagnation easily produces heat, as shown in previous cases. This is known as heat from constraint. This patient has obvious heat symptoms with sweating, meaning that the heat is severe enough to force out the body fluids. The patient has a dry throat, is thirsty, and wants to drink, indicating that some damage has been done to the body fluids.

Fig. 1

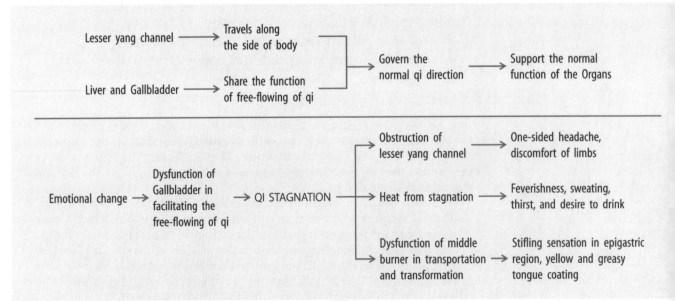

The free-flowing of qi also regulates the digestive function in the middle burner, thus qi stagnation in the lesser yang can influence the Stomach and Spleen. In this case the patient has a normal appetite so the function of the middle burner is still virtually unaffected. However, she has a stifling sensation after eating sweet foods, and the tongue coating is thick and greasy. This implies a slight accumulation of dampness, but the Spleen function is only mildly affected.

In Chinese medicine different tastes of food may affect different Organs if the taste is too strong or the Organ too weak. Sweet food readily gives rise to dampness and heat and impairs the function of the Stomach and Spleen. Hot, spicy food produces Heart fire. Very sour food injures the Liver.

The dark red tongue indicates that stagnant qi has transformed into heat, which is also shown by the dry, yellow coating. The coating is also thick and greasy, indicating the presence of dampness. The sunken, wiry pulse indicates qi stagnation.

Pattern of disease

This is both an interior and a channel-collateral pattern. The emotional change followed by qi stagnation inside the body has thus influenced the channel and Gallbladder.

The stagnant qi has already transformed into heat, making it a heat pattern.

The pattern is excessive because the history of this episode is short and there are no symptoms suggesting deficiency of the antipathogenic factors.

Additional notes

1. Is there an exterior pattern in this case?

According to basic Chinese medical theory, the channels are part of the superficial tissues. A problem may be localized to a channel where it is known as a channel-collateral disorder, or it may be part of a more general internal problem which has caused symptoms in the channel. In this case the emotional change has disturbed the qi activity and caused obstruction of the channel. The main complaint is headache, the site of disease being the channel and the Gallbladder. In this case the main problem is interior, the channel disorder being secondary.

2. Is the Liver involved in this case?

Emotional change is the principal cause of disease in this case, leading to dysfunction in the free-flowing of qi. This is usually regarded as a Liver disorder, but in this patient there are no symptoms associated with the Liver. The symptoms of pain along the course of the channel and the heat from constraint point to the Gallbladder. The Liver and Gallbladder have a close relationship, the Gallbladder assisting the Liver in encouraging the free-flow of qi. In this case only the function of the Gallbladder and lesser yang channel has been disturbed.

3. Does the left-sided chest pain indicate Heart qi deficiency or Heart blood stasis?

The symptoms are very mild and there are no other problems relating to the Heart such as palpitations, anxiety, dyspnea, or a stifling sensation in the chest. In this case there is merely a mild dysfunction of the qi in the chest as a result of the impairment to the free-flowing of qi.

Conclusion

1. According to the eight principles:
   Interior and channel-collateral combination, heat and excessive pattern.
2. According to etiology:
   Emotional change.
3. According to qi, blood, and body fluid theory:
   Qi stagnation transforming into heat.
4. According to channels and collaterals:
   Heat from constraint in the lesser yang channel.
5. According to Organ theory:
   Dysfunction of the Gallbladder in facilitating the free-flow of qi.

Treatment principle	1. Regulate the qi of the Gallbladder. 2. Remove the heat. 3. Remove the obstruction from the channel and alleviate pain.
Selection of points	G-8 *(shuai gu)* on right side *tai yang* (M-HN-9) on right side G-20 *(feng chi)* on right side G-34 *(yang ling quan)* on right side TB-7 *(hui zong)* on both sides LI-4 *(he gu)* on both sides K-7 *(fu liu)* on both sides S-36 *(zu san li)* on left side Sp-6 *(san yin jiao)* on left side
Explanation of points	G-8 *(shuai gu)* soothes the Liver qi and removes obstruction from the Gallbladder and Liver channels. It also removes heat from the lesser yang Organ and channel. When obstruction of these channels or stagnation in these Organs leads to lateral head symptoms, this is the primary point to use. It is a good point for alleviating pain. *tai yang* (M-HN-9) is mainly used as a local point to remove the symptoms in the temporal region and around the eye. It regulates qi and blood and alleviates pain. G-20 *(feng chi)* arrests both external and internal wind, removes obstruction from the channel, and promotes function in the eyes. In this case it is used on only one side to remove the obstruction from the lesser yang channel. G-34 *(yang ling quan)* is the lower sea point of the Gallbladder and is effective in removing heat due to stagnation from the Organ. It also strengthens Liver function and can be used when there are middle burner symptoms caused by disorder of the Liver or Gallbladder such as nausea, vomiting, or abdominal discomfort. S-36 *(zu san li)* regulates the Spleen and Stomach and promotes the body's resistance. In this case there are already some mild middle burner symptoms indicating a tendency for wood to invade earth. The point is used with an even technique to promote the function of the middle burner and prevent the invasion by wood. Sp-6 *(san yin jiao)* is used because of the presence of heat from stagnation. It promotes the yin aspect of the body and will therefore tend to clear heat and prevent consumption of body fluids. TB-7 *(hui zong)* is the accumulating point of the hand lesser yang channel and is effective in removing obstruction from the channel and alleviating pain. It is an important point in the treatment of lesser yang headache. LI-4 *(he gu)* is a point on the hand yang brightness channel and is used to prevent symptoms from reaching this channel. The patient complains of sweating and feeling hot; this point is chosen to clear the heat and also to help remove the discomfort in the yang brightness Organ. K-7 *(fu liu)* is the river point of the Kidney channel and is effective in nourishing the yin and removing heat. It is especially important to use this point when the symptoms indicate injury to the body fluids and the patient continues to sweat.
Combination of points	G-8 *(shuai gu)*, TB-7 *(hui zong),* and G-34 *(yang ling quan)* are all points on the lesser yang channels, but are located on the head, arm, and leg respectively. They all remove heat from stagnation and regulate the qi of the channel, thus this formula can be used to remove symptoms from both the lesser yang Organ and channel.

LI-4 *(he gu)* and K-7 *(fu liu)* is a combination that is traditionally used for treating abnormal sweating. It is also effective in nourishing the yin and clearing heat.

Laterality

Because this is in part a channel-level problem and the symptoms are unilateral, local points are used on the affected side. G-34 *(yang ling quan)* is a distal point on the affected channel, so it is also needled on the ipsilateral side. TB-7 *(hui zong)* is used to relieve obstruction from the hand lesser yang channels. Needling both the healthy and affected sides gives a greater effect. The systemic effects of LI-4 *(he gu)* and K-7 *(fu liu)* are very important here, and these points may accordingly be needled bilaterally because they are used for removing heat, nourishing the body fluids and soothing spontaneous sweating. S-36 *(zu sanli)* and Sp-6 *(san yin jiao)* are helping points. In order to reduce the number of needles, they can be chosen only on the healthy side.

Follow-up

The patient was treated only twice, on consecutive days. The headache disappeared and the sweating, feeling of heat, and discomfort in the chest were also relieved. The patient felt very relaxed after treatment and his mood became normal. The tongue coating became thin and white. The patient was rechecked after three and five months, but there was no recurrence of the headaches.

CASE 14: **Male, age 34**

Main complaint

Headache

History

Two weeks ago the patient was exposed to wind and cold and developed a headache. The pain was centered in three areas: the medial extremity of both eyebrows, the bridge of the nose, and the occipital region. The nape of the neck and the upper back were also stiff.

Later, pain also developed on the right side of the head. The pain is now worse than before and is continuous, the patient becoming nauseous when the pain is severe. Analgesics have had no effect. Whenever the patient goes out in the cold the pain intensifies. There is sensitivity and tenderness in the frontal region, the right side of the head, and the occipital region.

Tongue

Body is normal, coating is white

Pulse

Sunken, slightly slow, and forceful

Analysis of symptoms

1. Headache—obstruction of the channels.
2. Pain intensifies with exposure to cold—
    constriction of the channels by pathogenic cold.
3. Severe pain leading to nausea—reversal of Stomach qi.
4. White tongue coating—cold pattern.
5. Pulse is sunken, forceful, and slightly slow—stagnation of qi in the channels.

Basic theory of case

In Chinese medicine the headache caused by external pathogenic factors is called *tóu fēng* (literally 'head wind'). The migraine caused by external pathogenic factors is called *piān tóu fēng* ('lateral head wind').

The most common causes of head wind are wind-cold, wind-dampness, and wind-heat. These types of headache are characterized by rapid onset, history of exposure to pathogenic factors, and sensitivity to changes in the weather. Wind is common to all three types, as it is a yang pathogenic factor which always attacks the yang aspects of the body such as the head.

The symptoms of head wind are different from headache caused by other exterior patterns which involve the entire surface of the body. This is because the pathogenic factors are retained in the head alone, causing poor circulation of qi and blood and reducing the ability to exchange turbid and clear qi in the head. This is therefore a channel-collateral pattern. Another difference between these two patterns is that head wind can be very painful and last from one day to several weeks, while the purely exterior pattern will have a much shorter history.

Cause of disease

Pathogenic wind and cold

Before onset the patient was exposed to wind and cold; moreover the pain is aggravated by exposure to cold air. These symptoms indicate invasion by pathogenic wind and cold.

Site of disease

Channels

The pain is limited to three regions on the head: between the eyebrows, the bridge of the nose, and the back of the head and nape of the neck. This essentially traces the pathway of the foot greater yang Bladder channel. However, the pain later moves to the right side of the head, indicating that the lesser yang channel is also involved. There are no obvious symptoms related to any of the Organs except nausea, which will be explained later.

Pathological change

This patient has a clear history of exposure to cold wind and the pain is closely related to the weather. These symptoms are powerful evidence to suggest that the patient is suffering from exposure to pathogenic cold and wind which have obstructed the qi circulation in the channels on the head and caused headache. Because the channels are constricted by cold, further exposure to cold intensifies the pain, which is also aggravated by palpation of the affected areas. These symptoms together prove that the problem is one of excess.

The foot greater yang channel begins at the inner canthus of the eye, ascending by the medial extremity of the eyebrow over the head and down the nape, then traveling down the back to the legs and feet. The foot lesser yang Gallbladder channel governs the sides of the head, body, and legs, positioned between the yin and yang aspects. The pathogenic factors initially attacked the greater yang channel, the obstruction here causing the early symptoms. The pain then spread to attack the lesser yang channel, thus proceeding from the exterior toward the interior.

Nausea is a common symptom of reversal of the Stomach qi. This patient has nausea when the pain is severe, but he does not complain of any other digestive symptoms. Therefore we cannot yet diagnose a middle burner disorder. However, the course of the pathogenic factors is plain to see, as the greater yang and lesser yang channels have already been influenced, and now the nausea is the first sign that the yang brightness is in danger of being affected. The nausea is not continuous, so the extent of the disruption of the yang brightness is not yet significant. If the condition is allowed to develop, however, it could transform into a middle burner disorder.

The tongue body is normal because the pathogenic factors have as yet failed to penetrate to the interior. The white tongue coating reflects the presence of cold. The slow pulse also suggests a cold pattern, while the forceful nature of the pulse indicates that the antipathogenic factor is strong.

Fig. 2

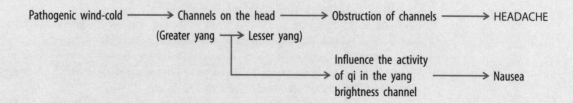

Pattern of disease

This is a channel-collateral pattern because the disorder was caused by an invasion of the channels by pathogenic factors.

Because the pathogenic factors are wind and cold, the symptom of severe pain is aggravated by cold, the tongue coating is white, and the pulse is slow, all of these symptoms indicate a cold pattern.

Because the pathogenic factors are strong and the antipathogenic factor is unaffected, this patient's pattern of disease is one of excess.

Additional notes

Why is the pulse sunken?

The patient does not have an interior pattern. The sunken pulse may have been present before onset, or it may represent the cold constricting the channels, but it does definitely show that the pattern of disease is not in the exterior, as then the pulse would be floating.

Conclusion

1. According to the eight principles:
   Channel-collateral, cold, and excessive pattern.
2. According to etiology:
   Invasion by pathogenic wind and cold.
3. According to channels and collaterals:
   Obstruction of the greater yang and lesser yang.
4. According to qi, blood, and body fluids:
   Channel qi stagnation.

Treatment principle

1. Remove the pathogenic wind and cold.
2. Relieve the obstruction in the channels and collaterals.
3. Alleviate the pain.

Selection of points

B-2 *(zan zhu)*
B-10 *(tian zhu)*
Ashi point on right side

Explanation of points

B-2 *(zan zhu)* removes obstruction, including that of wind, from the entire length of the channel and regulates the circulation of local qi and blood. This point also alleviates pain.

B-10 *(tian zhu)* is used to remove the symptoms of both the exterior pattern and the channel-collateral pattern. It is especially effective for problems of the neck and occipital region.

The combination of a point on the forehead, B-2 *(zan zhu),* and the neck, B-10 *(tian zhu),* ensures a strong treatment for the greater yang channel.

Ashi point: This point is selected by palpation. The most painful point will be punctured using a reducing method.

Note that this case is a good example of how acupuncture alone (without moxibustion) can successfully treat invasion of wind-cold. It is especially effective in cases with a short history.

Follow-up

After the first treatment the patient felt instant improvement in the areas of the eyebrows and back of the head. The following day the same points were used. After this treatment the headache was completely gone.

CASE 15: **Female, age 29**

Main complaint

Headache

History

The patient has a recurrent history of forehead pain of over ten years' duration. Over the years the pain has gradually become more severe. When the headaches began there was no obvious cause. In the last year the headaches have become much more frequent and severe. The accompanying symptoms in the head region are dizziness and a feeling of cold. The patient always wears a hat, even during the summer, because of sensitivity to cold. She also complains of a sticky white discharge from the nose and nasal obstruction. (Eight years ago X-rays revealed chronic sinusitis.) She has been treated with Western drugs and Chinese herbs, but the only result was temporary relief from the pain. The frequency of headaches has remained unchanged.

At present the patient has a very bad headache which has caused insomnia and loss of appetite for the past few days. She has no desire to drink and her urination is normal. She passes two loose, unformed stools per day. Her complexion is slightly pale.

Tongue

Slightly red body (i.e., normal), tongue coating is white

Pulse

Sunken and forceless

Analysis of symptoms

1. Forehead headache—obstruction of the channels.

2. Accompanied by a feeling of cold—yang deficiency.

3. Dizziness—failure of the clear yang to rise.

4. Lack of thirst, unformed stools—cold pattern.

5. Pale face, white tongue coating—cold pattern.

6. Sunken and forceless pulse—deficiency of the antipathogenic factor.

Basic theory of case

There is a famous saying, "The head is the meeting place of yang." This statement has two different meanings: first, the clear yang accumulates in the head (see the chapter on dizziness), and second, all of the yang channels meet in the head.

The hand greater yang Small Intestine channel begins on the hand and travels up to the face and ear. A branch of the hand greater yang connects with the origin of the foot greater yang Bladder channel at the inner canthus. The foot greater yang ascends over the forehead to the top of the head where it enters the brain via a collateral, then descends down to the nape, divides into two branches, and travels down the back and legs. Thus symptoms which involve the top of the head, nape, and back are associated with a greater yang disorder.

The hand yang brightness Large Intestine channel travels up the arm to the neck and face where it ends at the side of the nose. The foot yang brightness Stomach channel begins at this point, travels up the side of the nose, moves laterally and then down the cheek, around the mouth along the mandibular bone, then moves up in front of the ear to the forehead. Therefore the symptoms related to the forehead are associated with a yang brightness disorder.

The part of the hand lesser yang channel which is on the head is situated mainly around the ear. At the outer canthus it connects with the foot lesser yang Gallbladder channel. From here the foot lesser yang ascends to the lateral side of the head, moves behind the ear to the neck and back again across the lateral aspect of the head. Hence the symptoms which emerge on the lateral aspect of the head are primarily associated with a lesser yang disorder.

The governing vessel is regarded as the 'sea of yang'. It travels up the spinal column, through the center of the nape to the head, then continues along the midline of the head to the bottom of the nose. Symptoms which occur in this area are associated with the governing vessel.

Cause of disease

Pathogenic cold

The patient has a total intolerance to cold. She must wear a hat to prevent any aggravation of her problem. The severe pain and white nasal discharge further confirm that the pathogenic factor is cold.

Site of disease

Channels

The pain affects many of the channels on the head. The yang brightness channel is affected most severely because of the site of the pain.

Pathological change

Headache which is caused by an invasion of pathogenic factors is called head wind (see previous case). This patient's symptoms are caused by pathogenic cold. The yang brightness governs the forehead. When cold primarily invades the yang brightness channel the pain begins in this region. The obstruction of the channels impedes the circulation of qi and blood and disturbs the exchange of clear yang and turbid yin. The clear yang is unable to reach the head and dizziness results.

The nasal obstruction may result from two possible causes. First, the cold has attacked the nose which is the opening of the Lung. This disrupts the dispersal of Lung qi leading to nasal malfunction. Second, the yang brightness channel helps promote and support the nasal functions. If cold invades this channel, the nose will lose this support and cause nasal obstruction and/or discharge. This case can be attributed to the second cause inasmuch as there is an absence of any Lung symptoms such as copious nasal discharge, reduction in the sense of smell, or severe nasal obstruction.

The patient complains of oversensitivity to cold in the head region even in the warm summer months. This proves that the patient cannot resist the pathogenic cold and needs a hat to protect herself from the cold.

The poor appetite and insomnia are closely related to the headache as they are a direct result of the pain; hence these two symptoms are of no special pathological significance.

The pale face and white tongue coating both indicate the presence of cold in the body. The sunken and forceless pulse suggest that the antipathogenic factor is deficient.

Pattern of disease

This patient has a combination of interior and channel-collateral patterns. The pathogenic cold has obstructed the channels on the head, which represents the channel-collateral pattern. The deficiency of antipathogenic factor represents the interior pattern.

The patient has a cold feeling on the head, no desire to drink, loose stools, pale face, and white tongue coating, all of which confirm the presence of cold.

In this case there is a combination of excessive and deficiency patterns. Excess is indicated by the obstruction of the channels which is causing the pain, while the deep and forceless pulse indicates deficiency of the antipathogenic factor.

Additional notes

1. Is there enough evidence to prove that the headache was caused by an invasion of pathogenic factors?

Although this patient has a clear feeling of cold on her head, there is no history of exposure to cold. In general, an obvious history of exposure to pathogenic factors is important when diagnosing an exterior disorder. But in clinical practice the etiological differentiation can isolate the significant symptoms without obvious causes. For example, aversion to cold and fever indicate wind-cold, while fever with sweating, slight aversion to cold, and a floating, rapid pulse indicate wind-heat. In this case the extreme sensitivity to cold on the head confirms that the problem must be related to cold in the environment, even though the patient is unaware of any obvious overexposure to cold.

2. What evidence is there of an interior deficiency pattern?

We know that the antipathogenic factor is deficient owing to the sunken and forceless pulse. However, the category of antipathogenic factor deficiency is very broad. In this case the pale face, recurrent onset, and cold feeling on the head even in summer all confirm the existence of yang deficiency. The fact that the patient

Fig. 3

needs a hat during the summer when the environmental yang is abundant shows that the yang deficiency is severe.

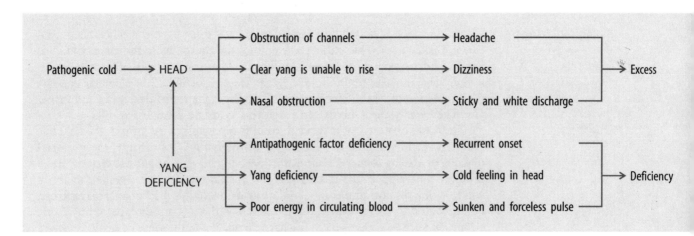

3. Can pathogenic factors stay in the channel to cause a long-term headache?

Usually external pathogenic factors will, if they persist for some time, travel into the body and give rise to an interior pattern, changing from cold to heat. So why has the cold remained in the channel for such a long time in this case?

In fact, this patient's headache was not continuous over the course of the past ten years. The yang deficiency allowed the recurrent invasion of pathogenic factors, but each time the cold did not remain very long. Therefore this is not a case of pathogenic cold obstructing a channel continuously for ten years.

4. Is there a heat pattern in this case?

When a patient has nasal obstruction and discharge, the pattern can be judged by the thickness and color of the discharge. If the discharge is clear, watery, or white, a cold pattern is evident. On the other hand, a thick and yellow discharge would indicate the presence of a heat pattern. This patient's discharge is white but sticky and thick. As there is no other evidence of heat, we should disregard the clinical significance of its thick and sticky qualities.

Conclusion

1. According to the eight principles:
   Channel-collateral and interior pattern, cold pattern with a combination of excess and deficiency; the main problem is excess, but there is also some yang deficiency.

2. According to etiology:
   Invasion by wind-cold.

3. According to channels and collaterals:
   Obstruction of the yang brightness channel, however the governing vessel and greater yang channel have also been affected.

Treatment principle

1. Expel the wind-cold.
2. Remove the obstruction from the channels.
3. Tonify the yang.

Selection of points
Prescription one

si shen cong (M-HN-1)
B-2 *(zan zhu)*
G-20 *(feng chi)*

Prescription two	GV-23 *(shang xing)* G-12 *(wan gu)* GV-20 *(bai hui)*

For both prescriptions moxa was applied for thirty minutes after needling was completed.

Explanation of points

si shen cong (M-HN-1): This group of points is used to remove the obstruction from the channels on the top of the head. Their selection in this case is mainly due to their suitability for the headache, but they also help to calm the patient's spirit.

B-2 *(zan zhu)* removes wind and promotes the function of the eye. It is located on each side of *yin tang* (M-HN-3). As there are two needles, their local effect will be stronger than needling *yin tang* (M-HN-3) alone.

G-20 *(feng chi)* removes the pathogenic wind and obstruction from the channel and forehead.

GV-23 *(shang xing)*: The main functions of this point are to remove wind and promote the yang qi in the head. Because this patient is suffering from yang deficiency, a point selected on the governing vessel near the forehead will serve the dual purpose of tonifying the yang and removing the wind. This point also has a favorable effect on the nose.

G-12 *(wan gu)* is chosen for its ability to remove the pathogenic factors and alleviate pain. It removes obstruction from the channels that traverse the forehead and face and is therefore used for treating pain in the forehead and facial paralysis.

GV-20 *(bai hui)* can remove local obstruction from the head and raise the yang to relieve the feelings of cold. The use of moxa at this point has a profound effect on the yang qi.

Clinically some lesser yang channel points are commonly used for treating yang brightness headache. The theoretical explanation for this is that the lesser yang channels also travel to the forehead. The present case illustrates this use of the points.

Follow-up

The patient received four treatments every other day with the first group of points. Although the headache was much improved, the extreme sensitivity to cold remained unchanged. The second prescription was then used everyday for three weeks (except Sunday). The second prescription utilized only four needles. Because the patient had a combination of excess and deficiency, this change was made to help protect the yang qi from the effect of too many needles. The symptoms gradually disappeared to the extent that the patient gave up wearing a hat, even though it was late autumn.

Both of these prescriptions contain points which are located on the head. In this case the local application of moxa was of paramount importance. Because the intense cold had been retained in the head region, the main thrust of the treatment was in the local area and short-range distal points like G-12 *(wan gu)* and G-20 *(feng chi)*.

CASE 16: **Male, age 32**

Main complaint

Headache

History

The patient has a seven year history of headaches, dating from an injury suffered when he fell from a height and struck the back of his head. He was unconscious for a short time, and upon regaining consciousness had severe headache and dizziness. The diagnosis at that time was cerebral concussion and he was treated symptomatically. After recovering he had only occasional occipital headaches.

Six months ago while he was working extremely hard without adequate rest the headaches became more frequent and severe. They were always occipital and he felt that the pain was similar to that which he experienced at the time of the injury. He also had dizziness, insomnia, and general lassitude. He returned to the hospital where he was diagnosed with sequelae from the head injury. At present the patient complains that reading causes the symptoms to become very severe and his concentration is impaired. His appetite, bowel movements, and urine are normal. His complexion is sallow and dry.

Tongue

The body is slightly red with obvious ecchymosis at the extreme tip. The coating is normal.

Pulse

Sunken and slightly thin

Analysis of symptoms

1. Headache—obstruction of the channels.
2. History of trauma—blood stasis.
3. Headache with dizziness—malnourishment of the head.
4. Lassitude with insomnia—malnourishment of the spirit.
5. Sallow complexion—blood is unable to nourish the face.
6. Ecchymosis on the tongue—blood stasis.
7. Sunken pulse—interior pattern.

Basic theory of case

In Chinese medicine the Heart stores consciousness, emotional response, and thought. In other words, the Heart 'houses the spirit.' The brain is also considered to be closely associated with these functions.

According to ancient knowledge of anatomy, the brain is known as the sea of marrow and is formed from the same tissue as the bone marrow. The Kidney controls the bones and produces the marrow, thus the Kidney essence produces and supports the marrow which includes the bone marrow, spinal cord, and brain. There is thus a close relationship between the brain and the Kidney.

In terms of physiological function the head and brain are known as the palace of the clear yang, the meeting place of yang, and the storehouse of intelligence and clear thought *(jīng míng)*. The head is therefore the place which forms the focal point for the yang qi, which is essential for efficient cerebral function. The brain plays an important role in maintaining consciousness and in all mental processes.

In Chinese medicine mental function is subdivided into five types, *shén, hún, yì, pò* and *zhì*:

Shén (or spirit) is the essential soul, spirit, or psyche of the individual.
Hún (ethereal soul) is the life-giving force which exists while the body is alive.
Yì (intention or reflection) means intelligent thought.
Pò (courage or daring) means emotional strength.
Zhì (will) means ability to judge.

These five aspects are associated respectively with the Heart, Liver, Spleen, Lung, and Kidney. Psychological function in Chinese medicine is therefore related to all five yin Organs. The spirit is mainly controlled by the Heart and brain, assisted by the other Organs. *See Fig. 4.*

Cause of disease

Blood stasis

This patient's headache was caused by traumatic injury. The tongue shows ecchymosis which indicates that the trauma has caused damage to the channels and vessels on the head, leading to poor circulation and blood stasis.

Fig. 4

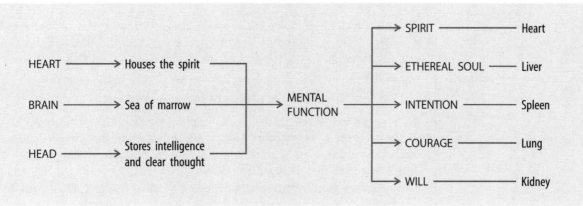

Site of disease	Channels

The injury occurred on the back of the head causing obstruction of the channels in the occipital area.

Pathological change

In our discussion of basic theory we mentioned that the brain is associated with the spirit. After head injury the normal psychological function can be disturbed in various ways. In this case the patient lost consciousness after the injury, indicating that the exchange between the clear yang and turbid yin in the head was impaired. The clear yang could not ascend to support the head and the normal brain function was thereby disturbed.

After a short time the patient regained consciousness but was left with recurrent headaches. The clear yang was able to rise to support the head, thus consciousness was restored, but the obstruction of qi and blood in the channels and collaterals remained, giving rise to recurrent headaches. After a period of time this type of obstruction may improve and disappear, or alternatively may progress to blood stasis. Factors influencing the outcome include the strength of the antipathogenic factor and also the treatment which the patient receives. Other factors such as stress, weather change, or adverse environmental factors may also affect the outcome.

This patient has blood stasis. For the past six months he has worked too hard and has consumed the yang qi and yin blood in the body. His sleep has been inadequate, which has prevented the replenishment of qi and blood. Previously he had slight impairment of qi and blood circulation, but this has now become severe, and the headaches are consequently more frequent. Qi is consumed by both mental and physical activity, but Spleen qi is mainly used for physical activity. Mental activity consumes the qi of the Heart, including the brain, so the headache is worse when the patient reads or engages in mental work. The qi circulation in the channels is poor and this in turn interferes with the rising of the clear yang, resulting in dizziness.

The sallow face indicates that nourishment is abnormal, the cause being the same as that which gave rise to the headaches. The general lassitude and insomnia indicate malnourishment of the spirit and blood stasis. The ecchymosis on the tip of the tongue shows blood stasis. The sunken pulse indicates an interior disorder. It is thin because there is malnourishment of the vessels.

Pattern of disease

There is no history of invasion by pathogenic factors, but there is a history of trauma. The injury to the head is inside; this is accordingly an interior pattern.

There is blood stasis present, but no obvious pattern of either cold or heat.

The headache is caused by obstruction of the channels with blood stasis, an excessive pattern.

Additional notes

1. What is the evidence to support a diagnosis of injury to the channels and collaterals?

There is a history of injury but the skin has not been broken. The channels and collaterals can be injured by severe force even when the skin is unbroken. The primary evidence for this aspect of the diagnosis is the lack of headaches prior to the injury.

2. How long has there been stasis of blood in this case?

Blood stasis in Chinese medicine can imply poor blood circulation, not necessarily the presence of thrombosis. (Where an embolism or thrombosis is present, of course, it will cause blood stasis.) In this case the blood stasis dates from the head injury when the circulation of blood was impaired. At that time the stagnation was mild, but has since gradually increased in severity, especially during the past six months.

3. Is there a pattern of deficiency in this case?

The patient has symptoms suggestive of blood deficiency, such as a sallow complexion, general lassitude, insomnia, and a thin pulse. He has a history of overwork and inadequate sleep which consumed the qi and blood of the body. In fact, the blood stasis in this case is the principal cause of the malnourishment of the body, thus the deficient pattern is relatively insignificant when compared to the blood stasis.

Conclusion

1. According to the eight principles:
   Channel-collateral and interior, neither heat nor cold, and excessive.
2. According to etiology:
   Blood stasis.
3. According to channels and collaterals:
   Obstruction of the channels mainly involving the governing vessel and the greater yang channels.

Treatment principle

1. Remove the blood stasis and obstruction from the channels.
2. Regulate the qi and alleviate the pain.

Selection of points

GV-16 *(feng fu)*
B-12 *(feng men)*
B-10 *(tian zhu)*
SI-3 *(hou xi)*

Explanation of points

In this case the pain is mainly in the occipital region, indicating obstruction of the governing vessel and greater yang channels, so the points are chosen primarily from these channels.

GV-16 *(feng fu)* is useful for removing stagnation from the brain and improving the circulation of qi and blood. It is also indicated for removing stagnation from the channel. The words *feng fu* mean 'palace of wind' in Chinese, so this point also arrests wind, and is used in the treatment of dizziness as well as to calm the spirit.

B-12 *(feng men)* is situated on the upper back and is regarded as a near distal point for the removal of obstruction from the greater yang channel. It is also a good point for preventing invasion by external pathogenic factors.

B-10 *(tian zhu)* is able to expel wind and other external factors, and also alleviates pain. It is located on the neck where the clear yang and turbid yin pass, and is thus beneficial to the regulation of qi and blood circulation.

SI-3 *(hou xi)* is one of the eight confluent points and is associated with the governing vessel. Its use promotes the yang of the body and improves the function of the brain. This point is located on the hand greater yang channel, the qi of which resonates with that of the foot greater yang channel.

Combination of points

B-10 *(tian zhu)* and SI-3 *(hou xi)* is a combination of hand and foot greater yang points. One point is local to the occipital region, the other distal, and in combination they affect both the greater yang and governing vessels, thereby treating symptoms on the neck and occipital regions.

Follow-up

This patient was treated seven times on alternating days. After one treatment the headache improved but other symptoms, especially the dizziness, remained unchanged. After six sessions the headache disappeared and the dizziness improved. He was sleeping well, but still felt very tired.

He was then treated six more times, once every three days, at the end of which all symptoms had gradually disappeared. Two months later he had no further headaches.

CASE 17: **Female, age 29**

Main complaint

Migraine for five years

History

Five years ago the patient suffered from hepatitis and was jaundiced. She also complained of nausea, poor appetite, abdominal distention, and pain in the liver region. She simultaneously developed headache in the occipital region, which was continuous for one month. When she recovered from hepatitis all the symptoms disappeared except for the headache, which recurred on the right temporal area and was often induced by eating cheese or sweet foods. The headache was also aggravated by menstruation. The weather did not affect it in any way. The headache was very sharp, usually accompanied by nausea and vomiting, and the patient became hypersensitive to noise. The headache could last for a few hours or even a few days. The pain was sometimes relieved by analgesics.

In recent months the migraines have become more frequent. For the last seven days the patient suffered a continuous migraine which was not relieved by analgesics. She has abdominal distention, difficulty in sleeping, and no appetite. Bowel movements and urination are normal. Her menstrual cycle is extremely irregular. She is presently taking hormones in an attempt to regulate the cycle. In the last two years her body weight has increased markedly (over 15kg) even though she eats very little food.

Tongue

Body is normal in color, white, with a slightly thick coating

Pulse

Sunken, slightly wiry

Analysis of symptoms

1. Headache—obstruction of the channels.
2. Poor appetite, abdominal distention—
     retention of dampness in the middle burner.
3. Nausea and vomiting—reversal of Stomach qi.
4. Headache not affected by weather—no invasion by pathogenic factors.
5. Headache brought on by menstruation—
     poor circulation of qi and blood in the channels.
6. Thick, white tongue coating—retention of dampness.
7. Sunken pulse—interior disorder.

Basic theory of case

The consumption of food is an essential part of life, but improper food intake is also a well-known cause of disease. There are three components to this phenomenon: overeating or not eating enough, intake of unclean food, or overeating one type of food.

According to the five phase theory, the five yin Organs are associated with different tastes. A varied diet will properly nourish the five yin Organs, while overconsumption of a single kind of food may lead to an imbalance of yin and yang in the related Organ. If this continues for a long time, eventually a disease will emerge.

For example, sour food can nourish Liver qi, but too much of it will harm the Liver; sweet food can tonify the Spleen and Stomach, yet too much sweet food can injure them by upsetting the directional flow of qi in the middle burner; salty food can nourish the Kidney, however overconsumption of salty food will upset water metabolism in the Kidney. In addition, rich or greasy products like animal meats, animal fats, alcohol, and dairy products can lead to retention of damp-heat. This information may be of value to the therapist.

Cause of disease

Retention of dampness

The patient has a history of dampness being retained in the middle burner five years ago. She had severe nausea, poor appetite, and abdominal distention. The headache can also be traced back to this time. Sweet foods and cheese make the symptoms much worse, and the headache is accompanied by severe nausea or vomiting. The presence of the thick, white tongue coating is further evidence of retention of dampness.

Site of disease

Channels and middle burner

The headache always occurs on the right side of the head. Clearly there is obstruction of the channels here.

The headache is always accompanied by digestive problems, which indicates a middle burner disorder.

Pathological change

The initial cause of the headache is a little unusual. It began at the same time as the hepatitis, so does this necessarily mean that there is a close relationship between these two problems?

According to the patient's history, we know she had suffered from nausea, poor appetite, and abdominal distention which were all caused by retention of dampness in the Stomach and Spleen. Simultaneously the patient had a headache, which was attributed to dampness in the channel, the same cause as the symptoms in the middle burner. The foot greater yang channel passes through the occipital region, nape, and back, hence initially the greater yang channel was affected.

Dampness is very greasy by nature and is difficult to remove when it becomes established in the body. This explains the chronic, recurrent pattern of the disorder. Pathogenic factors have a tendency to move deeper into the body. This is demonstrated here by the pain moving from the occipital region (greater yang) to the right side of the head (lesser yang).

Because of the retention of dampness in the middle burner, foods which promote dampness will aggravate the symptoms. In this case, cheese and the overconsumption of sweet foods aggravate her headaches. The pain becomes more intense before her periods because this further weakens the circulation of qi and blood in the body. The environment has no influence on her headache because dampness has accumulated inside the body. The retention of dampness in the middle burner disturbs the directional flow of qi, causing nausea and vomiting.

The thick, white tongue coating indicates retention of dampness in the middle burner, the sunken pulse an interior disorder with poor qi circulation, and its wiry quality is associated with pain.

Fig. 5

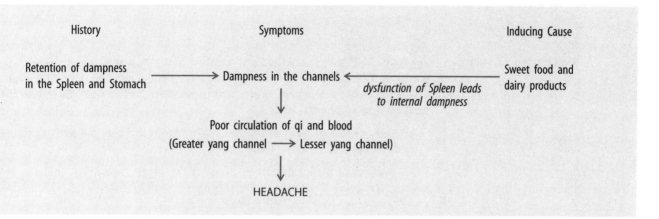

History	Symptoms	Inducing Cause
Retention of dampness in the Spleen and Stomach	→ Dampness in the channels ← *dysfunction of Spleen leads to internal dampness*	Sweet food and dairy products

Poor circulation of qi and blood
(Greater yang channel ——→ Lesser yang channel)

↓

HEADACHE

Pattern of disease	Combination of an interior with a channel-collateral pattern because the patient has retention of dampness in the middle burner and obstruction in the channel. The tongue coating is white and the pulse is not rapid, indicating a cold pattern. The pattern of disease is also excessive because both retention of dampness in the middle burner and obstruction of the lesser yang channel are excessive in nature.
Additional notes	1. Is there any blood stasis in this case? A typical dampness-type headache is heavy and dull, but here the pain is sharp which is normally a characteristic of blood stasis. How do we explain this? According to the symptoms and the pathological change we know the patient has severe retention of dampness, such as marked increase in weight and other symptoms of middle burner dysfunction. This is the initial cause of the poor circulation of qi and blood in the channels leading to sharp pain. But there are no other symptoms to indicate blood stasis. Moreover, neither the tongue nor pulse display symptoms of blood stasis. 2. Is there any Spleen deficiency? Dampness and sweet food can affect the transportive and transformative functions of the Spleen. Moreover, the patient's body weight is increasing although she eats very little food. The patient therefore does have a Spleen disorder, namely retention of dampness. However, this is not a type of deficiency and the symptoms will improve as the dampness is removed.
Conclusion	1. According to the eight principles: Interior and channel-collateral, cold, and excessive pattern. 2. According to etiology: Retention of dampness. 3. According to channels and collaterals: Obstruction of the lesser yang channel. 4. According to Organ theory: Retention of dampness in the Spleen and Stomach.
Treatment principle	1. Remove the dampness from the middle burner. 2. Resolve the obstruction of the lesser yang channel to alleviate the pain.
Selection of points	*tai yang* (M-HN-9) [right] G-20 *(feng chi)*

TB-5 *(wai guan)*
CV-12 *(zhong wan)*
Sp-9 *(yin ling quan)*
S-36 *(zu san li)*

Explanation of points

Tai yang (M-HN-9) is a good local point for removing obstruction and regulating the qi and blood and is commonly used for headache, dizziness, and some eye disorders. Because the pain in this case is on the right side only, this point is only used on the affected side.

G-20 *(feng chi)* removes pathogenic factors from the channel and regulates the qi and blood in the lesser yang channel.

TB-5 *(wai guan)* is the connecting point of the Triple Burner channel and is very good at removing obstruction from this channel. Thus it treats the head symptoms which are related to the lesser yang channel.

CV-12 *(zhong wan)* is used with even movement to regulate the qi in the middle burner and remove dampness.

Sp-9 *(yin ling quan)* removes dampness and tonifies the Spleen.

S-36 *(zu san li)* reinforces the function of the middle burner and regulates the qi.

Follow-up

The patient was treated twice per week for two weeks. After the first treatment the headache immediately disappeared, but it recurred mildly during the week with one six-hour bout. There was still mild nausea. The patient was then treated once a week for three weeks. After these treatments the digestive symptoms had disappeared, but occasionally she still had very slight headaches for short periods of time. Because her sleep was still unsound, GV-20 *(bai hui)* was added to the prescription and she was treated every other week for another four weeks. At this time she had very mild, temporary headaches only after working very hard. On follow-up six months later she reported no more bad headaches.

CASE 18: **Male, age 23**

Main complaint

Headache

History

The patient has a five-year history of recurrent headaches which have become more frequent and severe during the past year. There is no obvious precipitating factor and the headaches are unpredictable in onset. There is no association with changes in the weather. The pain is mainly on the forehead, eyebrows, and orbit, while the occiput feels stiff and tense. He has severe photophobia during the headaches, accompanied by violent nausea and vomiting, and his face becomes pale. The headaches last from 1-3 days during an attack. They interfere with sleep and affect the appetite. When he has no headache his appetite is good, but he often has a dry mouth and foul breath. His urine and bowels are normal.

Tongue

Slightly red tip; the body is soft and flabby with a thin, white, moist coating

Pulse

Sunken and thin

Analysis of symptoms

1. Recurrent headache—obstruction in the channels.
2. Symptoms unrelated to weather change—
     no invasion by external pathogenic factors.
3. Nausea and vomiting—reversal of Stomach qi.
4. Headache associated with pallor of the face—obstruction of the yang qi.
5. Foul breath—disruption of the descending function of the Stomach.

6. Flabby, soft tongue with moist, white coating—
   dysfunction of water metabolism due to yang qi deficiency.

7. Sunken, thin pulse—yang qi deficiency.

Basic theory of case

In Chinese medicine the head is the area in which the clear yang accumulates. If the clear yang cannot rise up to the head many problems can occur, such as dizziness and certain types of headache. The failure of the clear yang to rise may be attributed to either excess or deficiency.

In the case of deficiency, the yang qi is weak and this can result in either yang deficiency headache or qi deficiency headache. The excessive pattern is the result of pathological factors, usually retained dampness or phlegm, blocking the path of the clear yang.

One of the characteristics of headache due to retention of dampness is a widespread feeling of heaviness, implying that the dampness has blocked the channels and has also remained in the tissues, such as skin and muscle. Headache associated with phlegm is characterized by more localized symptoms. Phlegm often accumulates in the middle burner, resulting in reversal of Stomach qi, thus nausea and vomiting are commonly present.

In the clinical situation the picture may be complex with the presence of both excess and deficiency patterns; indeed, there may be both retention of dampness and accumulation of phlegm. It is therefore important to determine which patterns are present and to make out their relationship in order to ascertain the main cause of the headache.

Cause of disease

Phlegm

The headache has no relationship to changes in the weather and there is severe nausea and vomiting with pallor of the face. The flabby tongue, moist tongue coating, and sunken pulse all indicate retention of phlegm inside the body, obstructing qi and yang activity.

Site of disease

Channels and Stomach

The symptoms of each headache are very similar, always occurring at the same sites; this indicates obstruction of the channels.

The patient also experiences nausea and vomiting on each occasion, which suggests that the Stomach is involved.

Pathological change

The middle burner is the source of production of qi and blood and has an important role in the exchange of the clear and turbid qi. When phlegm accumulates in the Stomach the qi activity is obstructed and the normal ascending and descending of qi is impaired. The clear yang cannot ascend to the head and the turbid yin cannot descend.

The headache in this case is caused by accumulation of phlegm, which in turn affects the circulation of qi and blood in the head. The pain is mainly on the forehead, eyebrows, orbit, and occipital region, in other words the obstruction is on the yang brightness and greater yang channels, and both channels are affected simultaneously.

Because the middle burner qi is obstructed by phlegm, the Stomach qi reverses and causes nausea and vomiting. The yang qi is the force which circulates the blood. When it is obstructed during a severe headache, the blood cannot circulate efficiently, resulting in facial pallor.

The appetite is good when the headache is not present, but the patient has foul breath. This indicates that the accumulated phlegm is causing mild reversal of Stomach qi even when there is no headache.

The tongue body is flabby and soft and the coating is thin, white, and moist. These are symptoms of yang deficiency together with impairment of water metabolism. It can be seen in patterns of retention of cold and dampness as well as accumulation of phlegm. The sunken, thin pulse indicates yang qi deficiency.

Pattern of disease

This is a combination of a channel-collateral pattern and an interior pattern. There is obstruction of the head indicating a channel disorder, and retention of phlegm in the middle burner, an interior pattern.

This is also a cold pattern because there is both yang deficiency and accumulation of phlegm-cold.

This is likewise a combination of excess and deficiency patterns: phlegm obstructing the qi activity is a problem of excess, and there is also deficiency of yang qi.

Additional note

Is there a heat pattern in this case?

The patient has a dry mouth and the tip of the tongue is slightly red. While this could be explained in terms of heat, the subjective symptom of a dry mouth can also be due to lack of production of body fluids. In this case there is obstruction of the middle burner by phlegm retention causing yang qi deficiency, which in turn has led to a reduction in the production of body fluids.

The red tongue tip is not easily explained, but as there are no other symptoms relating to heat, it can be disregarded.

Conclusion

1. According to the eight principles:
   Channel-collateral and interior pattern, cold, and a combination of excess and deficiency patterns, the deficiency being within an excess.
2. According to etiology:
   Retention of phlegm.
3. According to channels and collaterals:
   Obstruction in the greater yang and yang brightness channels.
4. According to Organ theory:
   Retention of phlegm in the Stomach, yang qi deficiency.
5. According to yin-yang theory:
   Yang qi deficiency.

Treatment principle

1. Remove the phlegm and obstruction from the channels.
2. Regulate the qi of the middle burner.
3. Reinforce the yang qi.

Selection of points

G-14 *(yang bai)* and *yin tang* (M-HN-3), used alternately
B-10 *(tian zhu)*
LI-4 *(he gu)*
S-40 *(feng long)*
S-36 *(zu san li)*

Explanation of points

G-14 *(yang bai)* is a point on the Gallbladder channel but is also an important local point for yang brightness headache. It effectively regulates the qi and blood and improves the function of the eyes. It is effective for symptoms around the eyes, eyebrows, and forehead.

yin tang (M-HN-3) is a local point that is useful for removing obstruction and for alleviating pain. It is effective in treating forehead symptoms.

B-10 *(tian zhu)* regulates the qi in the foot greater yang channel, and expels pathogenic wind and alleviates pain. It is used for local pain and stiffness in the occipital region.

LI-4 *(he gu)* is very effective in alleviating pain and removing obstruction from the channels and collaterals. It is a classical distal point for yang brightness headache, and is also effective for relieving pain in the eyes.

S-40 *(feng long)* expels phlegm and calms the spirit, and removes obstruction from both the yang brightness channel and Organ.

S-36 *(zu san li)* regulates the Stomach and the Spleen and promotes the antipathogenic factor. It is also useful for removing obstruction from the channel. In this case it is used to harmonize the function of the middle burner, alleviate the nausea and vomiting, and reinforce the yang qi.

Combination of points

G-14 *(yang bai), yin tang* (M-HN-3), and LI-4 *(he gu)*: These three points are a small formula for treating yang brightness headache, a combination of local points with a distant point. G-14 *(yang bai)* and *yin tang* (M-HN-3) can be used together or alternately depending on the severity of the headache.

Follow-up

This patient was treated only four times in the course of a month, the second treatment being five days after the initial treatment session. He was treated again ten days later, and given a final treatment after a further interval of two weeks.

After one treatment he had mild discomfort on the head lasting one day, and between the second and third sessions he had one headache lasting six hours with very mild nausea. He had no further headaches after one month and was discharged. The patient was advised to return if the headaches recurred. After a period of nearly two years there was no report from the patient.

Diagnostic principles for headache

Headache as a symptom can appear in a multitude of ways. It can manifest in different areas of the head and be lateral, frontal, global, or just at the vertex. The type of pain can also vary. It can be continuous, episodic, throbbing, sharp, or distending. Sometimes the patient with headache will have accompanying symptoms like dizziness, nausea, or vomiting. However, no matter how complicated a headache may seem, the diagnosis is always made by applying the following two steps: 1) assess the cause of the disorder, and 2) determine the site of the disorder.

Assessing the cause of disorder

The causes of headache can be divided into two broad groups, invasion of an external pathogenic factor, or interior dysfunction.

The primary characteristics of headache caused by an external pathogenic factor are rapid onset, and severe and continuous pain. Most of the headaches within this category are excessive in nature.

An interior dysfunction can also cause headache. For example, either internal phlegm, blood stasis, or an Organ disorder can cause a disharmony between qi and blood or yin and yang which results in headache. The primary characteristics of this type of headache are slow onset and sometimes episodic pain which tends to be not too severe. The pattern can be excessive, deficient, or a combination of the two.

More detail about the two types of headache is provided in Figure 6.

Pathology of headache

There are several different types of headache in Chinese medicine.

1. Wind-cold

The greater yang channel is the most vulnerable to attack by wind-cold. This pattern will exhibit pain or soreness in the upper back and neck. Pain from wind-cold is continuous because the cold is constricting the channels. Further exposure to cold will often aggravate the symptoms.

Fig. 6

HEADACHE CAUSED BY INVASION OF PATHOGENIC FACTORS

CAUSE	CHARACTER OF HEADACHE	ACCOMPANYING SYMPTOMS
Wind-cold	Continuous, whole head	Fever & aversion to cold, often affects whole head, no sweating or thirst, thin, white tongue coating, stiffness on the nape & upper back, floating & tight pulse, aggravated by cold
Wind-heat	Severe	Hot sensation or even explosive headache, high fever, red face and eyes, thirst with desire to drink, yellow urine, constipation, red tongue, yellow coating, rapid or floating pulse
Wind-dampness	Distending or heavy sensation	Aversion to cold, fever, heaviness about body or limbs, stifling sensation in the chest, loose stools, white & greasy tongue coating, soft pulse

HEADACHE CAUSED BY INTERIOR DYSFUNCTION

CAUSE	CHARACTER OF HEADACHE	ACCOMPANYING SYMPTOMS
Preponderance of yang	Distending, can have severe pain accompanied by dizziness, recurrent onset	Irritability or restlessness, insomnia, red complexion, bitter taste, tinnitus, or unstable walking with heavy feeling in the head and light on the foot, yellow tongue coating, rapid pulse
Qi deficiency	Mild and chronic, alternately better or worse from time to time, worsens with physical movement	General lassitude or fatigue, poor appetite, pale complexion, pale tongue and white coating, forceless pulse
Brain essence deficiency	Mild with empty feeling and long history, very poor memory	Soreness and weakness in the lower back and knee joints, cold appearance and limbs, lassitude, insomnia, tinnitus or seminal emotion or involuntary emotion, little tongue coating, thin and forceless pulse
Retention of dampness and phlegm	Accompanied by dizziness or heavy sensation, blurred spirit	Stifling sensation in the chest, epigastric distention, poor appetite, nausea, vomiting, loose stools, white, thick & greasy tongue coating, slippery pulse
Blood stagnation	Chronic with fixed site, sharp or throbbing pain, or traumatic headache	Mild general symptoms or absence of any general discomfort, dark tongue or with ecchymosis, thin or choppy pulse

2. Wind-heat

This group includes summerheat and fire. Because heat rises it naturally attacks the head where it disturbs the balance of qi and blood circulation. Often this will cause severe pain and stimulate other symptoms of heat in the body.

3. Wind-dampness

Dampness is turbid and heavy, hence it usually blocks the normal circulation of qi and blood in the channels. The patient will feel heaviness around the entire head. Some will have a feeling of heaviness together with a strong distending sensation around the entire head. If the dampness accumulates in the body and limbs, heaviness will be felt there too.

4. Preponderance of yang

There are two distinct types within this category. The first is pure excess, and the second is a combination of excess within a pattern of deficiency. A common feature of both is that heat rises up to disturb the qi and blood in the head. This often causes headache accompanied by vertigo.

5. Qi deficiency

When there is qi deficiency the circulation of qi and blood will become sluggish. The headache will vary in its intensity with the fluctuation in the level of qi deficiency. Any activity which consumes qi, e.g., thinking, physical exertion, etc., will tend to aggravate the headache.

6. Brain essence deficiency

In Chinese this is known as *suǐ hǎi bù chōng*. When the vital essence is deficient the brain will not be properly nourished, leading to a slowdown in mental acuity; symptoms like poor memory or poor concentration will emerge. The headache is usually a dull, mild background type of discomfort. In the clinic some patients will complain of an uncomfortable or empty feeling in the head.

7. Retention of phlegm and dampness

These are substantial pathogenic factors which can obstruct the proper circulation of qi and blood and block the rise of clear yang to the head. This type of headache is often characterized by a heavy sensation or dizziness. Sometimes there may also be drowsiness.

8. Blood stasis

Local physical trauma or injury can cause direct damage to a channel or vessel and lead to headache. (There are other causes of blood stasis as well.) When a headache is chronic and continuous in nature with a sharp or throbbing pain, then the primary cause will be blood stasis.

Determining the site of disorder

Fig. 7

The head has a close relationship with the Organs and channels of the body. Diagnosis can be made based upon the location of the headache and its accompanying symptoms. The following chart shows the associations between painful areas on the head and the affected channels.

AFFECTED CHANNEL	SITE OF PAIN
Greater yang channel	Occipital region, can affect neck and upper back
Yang brightness channel	Forehead
Lesser yang channel	One or both lateral sides of head, often focuses on temple region or around ear
Greater yin channel	Heavy or distending sensation around upper part of head
Lesser yin channel	Inside of head, affects teeth
Terminal yin channel	Vertex region

The three yang channel headaches have already been discussed in the previous cases. The pathology of the three yin channel headaches is discussed below.

The greater yin headache is primarily caused by a disorder of the foot greater yin channel. The pathogenic factor has affected the rising of clear yang and water metabolism, hence turbid yin accumulates in the head. The headache will display a heavy quality, particularly around the upper half of the head. Some patients will describe it as being like a wet bandage or towel wrapped around the head.

The foot lesser yin channel transfers vital essence upwards to the head where it nourishes the brain and teeth. (Teeth are regarded as the surplus of the bone.) If the problem is associated with the lesser yin channel, the headache will be described as deep inside, and will sometimes radiate to the teeth.

The foot terminal yin channel is associated with the vertex of the head where it meets the governing vessel. When the channel is disrupted by a pathogenic factor, the headache will affect the vertex of the head.

Disorders of the Organs can also cause headaches. In the clinical situation the most commonly affected Organs are the Liver, Spleen, and Kidney. The following chart shows the various patterns.

Fig. 8

AFFECTED YIN ORGAN	SYMPTOMS
LIVER	
Preponderance of Liver yang	Headache with vertigo, recurrent onset, often results from emotional change, irritability or restlessness, tinnitus, insomnia, unstable walking, soreness and weakness of the lower back and knees, red tongue, thin & yellow coating, thin & wiry pulse
Liver fire rising	Severe headache with onset often resulting from sudden anger or strong emotional change, irritability, bitter taste in mouth, thirst, severe insomnia, yellow urine, dry stool, red tongue, yellow, dry & thick coating, wiry & forceful pulse
SPLEEN	
Spleen qi deficiency	Mild headache, aggravated by physical activity, lassitude, poor appetite, abdominal distention, loose stools, pale tongue, white coating, forceless pulse
Spleen dysfunction caused by retention of dampness or phlegm	Headache with dizziness or heavy sensation, stifling sensation in the chest, epigastric distention, poor appetite, nausea, vomiting, loose stools, white, thick & greasy tongue coating, slippery pulse
KIDNEY	
Kidney essence deficiency	Headache with empty feeling in the head, very poor memory, loose teeth, tinnitus, alopecia, slow responses, hypofunction of sexual activity, or accompanied by other symptoms of Kidney yang or yin deficiency

The entire diagnostic procedure for headache is summarized in Figure 9.

HEADACHE

Is there a short history?

— Yes — Short history. Headache with exterior symptoms — Caused by Invasion of Pathogenic Factors

— No — Long history or recurrent onset. Headache without exterior symptoms — Caused by Interior Dysfunction

Caused by Invasion of Pathogenic Factors

Cause of disorder (according to etiology)

WIND-COLD
Continuous headache, worse with cold, aversion to cold, fever, thin and white tongue coating, floating and tight pulse

WIND-HEAT
Severe headache, hot sensation, thirst with desire to drink, red tongue, yellow coating, rapid pulse

WIND-DAMPNESS
Distending headache with heavy sensation, aversion to cold, fever, heaviness about body or limbs, suffocating sensation in the chest, white and greasy tongue coating, soft pulse

Site of disorder (according to channels and collaterals)

GREATER YANG CHANNEL
Occipital region, can affect nape and upper back

YANG BRIGHTNESS CHANNEL
Forehead

LESSER YANG CHANNEL
One or both lateral sides of head

GREATER YIN CHANNEL
Heavy or distending sensation around upper part of head

LESSER YIN CHANNEL
Inside of head, affects teeth

TERMINAL YIN CHANNEL
Vertex region

Caused by Interior Dysfunction

Cause of disorder (according to character of headache)

PREPONDERANCE OF YANG
Distending headache, perhaps severe pain, accompanied by dizziness, recurrent onset, often results from emotional change

QI DEFICIENCY
Mild and chronic headache, alternately better or worse, aggravated by physical activity

DAMPNESS AND PHLEGM
Headache with dizziness, or heavy sensation, blurred mind

BRAIN ESSENCE DEFICIENCY
Mild headache with empty feeling and long history, very poor memory

BLOOD STAGNATION
Chronic headache with sharp or throbbing pain, or traumatic headache

Site of disorder (according to Organ theory)

LIVER YANG PREPONDERANCE
Unstable walking, soreness and weakness in the lumbar region and knees, red tongue, thin and yellow coating, thin and wiry pulse

LIVER FIRE RAISING
Severe insomnia, yellow urine, dry stool, red tongue, yellow, dry and thick coating, wiry and forceful pulse

— LIVER

SPLEEN QI DEFICIENCY
Lassitude, poor appetite, abdominal distention, loose stool, pale tongue, white coating, forceless pulse

SPLEEN DYSFUNCTION caused by RETENTION OF DAMP-PHLEGM
Suffocating sensation in the chest, epigastric distention, poor appetite, nausea, vomiting, loose stool, white, thick and sticky tongue coating, slippery pulse

— SPLEEN

KIDNEY ESSENCE DEFICIENCY
Hypofunction of sexual activity, accompanied by Kidney yang or Kidney yin deficiency symptoms

— KIDNEY

CHANNEL OBSTRUCTION
Mild general symptoms or absence of any general discomfort, dark tongue or with ecchymosis, thready or hesitant pulse

— CHANNELS

Lower Back Pain

CASE 19: **Male, age 29**

Main complaint

Lower back pain

History

The patient has a two-year history of recurrent lower back pain. The main symptoms in the lower back are coldness, pain, and heaviness. The symptoms worsen on cloudy or cold days, and are alleviated by warmth. Sometimes the lower back pain radiates forward to cause discomfort in the lower abdominal area. The patient has no recollection of any obvious causative factors. He has a very slight reduction in appetite and is not thirsty. The urine is yellow and normal in quantity. He has a bowel movement only once every two or three days, the stools being normal. The patient has no problem with sleeping.

Tongue

Pale body, white, greasy coating

Pulse

Sunken, thin pulse

Analysis of symptoms

1. Lower back pain—obstruction of the channels.
2. Coldness, pain, and heaviness, all worsen with cold and improve with warmth—retention of pathogenic cold and dampness in the channels.
3. Normal quantity of urine, normal quality of stools—normal level of body fluids.
4. Pale tongue and white coating—cold pattern.
5. Thin pulse and greasy tongue coating—pathogenic dampness.

Basic theory of case

The theory of the channels and collaterals is very important in Chinese medicine. This theory is the most widely used concept in acupuncture because many disorders involve problems of the channels and collaterals. The system is a network of pathways for distributing qi and blood throughout the entire body, each channel and collateral having its unique route in the body. These routes all have connections with the Organs. In the clinical situation, diagnosis is based upon where the symptoms emerge and which channel or collateral is involved in that area. Diagnosis according to the channels and collaterals is therefore of great importance in Chinese medicine.

The superficial tissues are comprised of the skin, interstices and pores, channels and collaterals. When pathogenic factors invade the channels and collaterals, the disorder is classified as exterior in nature, although not necessarily as an exterior pattern. In Chinese medicine the requirements for diagnosing an exterior pattern are very strict. The mechanism is an invasion of the entire body surface, leading to stagnation of the protective qi. The symptoms must include feverishness and an aversion to cold; if these characteristics are absent, the condition cannot be called an exterior pattern.

When pathogenic factors invade the channels and collaterals the primary consequence will be obstruction of qi and blood. The patient will complain of local discomfort or pain, but there is an absence of aversion to cold and feverishness. In other words, although the site of disease is in the superficial tissues, the pathological change and symptoms of a disorder in the channels and collaterals are different from those of an exterior pattern. In order to avoid confusion, the term channel-collateral pattern will thus be utilized in this book.

Fig. 1

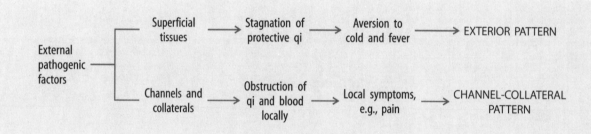

The pathogenic factors can also influence the Organs through the channels and collaterals. This creates a commonly seen mixture of interior-exterior disorder. We call this a combination channel-collateral and interior pattern.

Cause of disease

Damp-cold

The patient has lower back pain with symptoms of coldness and heaviness. These symptoms are strongly influenced by the environment and are relieved by warmth. The patient also has a greasy tongue coating and a thin pulse. All of these symptoms reflect the presence of dampness and cold.

Site of disease

Channels and collaterals

The patient has lower back pain which is aggravated by damp and cold weather. There is also pain along the course of the channel which radiates forward to the lower abdominal region. These symptoms indicate that the site of disease is in the channels and collaterals.

The patient's overall health is good, as indicated by his food intake, sleep pattern, and urinary habits. This generally healthy condition lends support to the diagnosis that the site of disease is the channels and collaterals.

Pathological change

Depending on the nature of the external factors involved, lower back pain (sometimes also involving lower limb pain) caused by pathogenic factors can display different symptoms.

Damp-cold is one of the most common combinations of pathogenic factors seen in the clinic. Both dampness and cold are yin pathogenic factors. Dampness is heavy, turbid, and has a tendency to migrate downwards. In the natural environment dampness will always accumulate on the ground or in areas close to ground level. In the body dampness likewise gathers in the lower aspects, e.g., the lower back and the lower limbs.

People may be predisposed to invasion by pathogenic dampness for various reasons. Some people live or work in damp and cold environments and hence suffer prolonged exposure to the pathogenic factors. Others who live in dry environments are at particular risk if they suddenly encounter damp and cold conditions, as they have very little resistance.

Dampness is heavy and cloying in nature, and obstructs the circulation of qi and blood. Heaviness is the main distinguishing feature of a damp disorder. Because it is a substantial pathogenic factor, dampness is very difficult to remove from the body. Damp disorders tend to persist for long periods of time, as in this case.

Although the original cause of the disorder here is unknown, the symptoms tell us there is damp-cold involvement, particularly the heavy sensation in the lower back, as well as the pain and cold. Based upon the area where the pain is located we also know which channels are involved: the governing vessel and foot greater yang Bladder channel. The governing vessel has a connection with the lower abdominal region. When there is retention of pathogenic factors in these two channels, obstruction of qi and blood will result. This explains why the patient has lower back pain with radiation into the lower abdomen.

Cold constricts the flow of qi and blood. When the body fails to receive yang support from the environment, the obstruction of the channels, and thus the lower back pain, become worse. Because warmth enhances the circulation of qi and blood, the lower back pain therefore improves with warmth.

Fig. 2

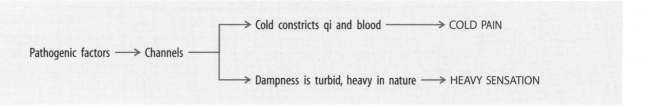

In this case the dampness and cold have been retained in the channels and collaterals. The penetration has not been deep, and the Organs are unaffected. This explains why the patient's general health is still good. Even though there is a slight decrease in appetite this is not a serious problem.

The tongue is pale and the coating is white because cold has constricted the flow of yang qi; the greasy tongue coating primarily indicates dampness. In general, a sunken pulse is a sign of an interior disorder, but in this case the sunken pulse is an indication of something quite different. The qi in the channels is compressed and constricted by pathogenic dampness and cold, thus the qi cannot rise to reach the superficial tissues. The thin nature of the pulse is a further indication of retention of dampness in the body.

Pattern of disease

This is a channel-collateral pattern because there is retention of damp-cold in the channels and collaterals.

A cold pattern is indicated by pain and coldness in the lower back, and by the patient's desire for warmth locally. There is a pale tongue with a white coating and an absence of thirst, all of which indicate retention of cold.

The pathogenic factors have been retained in the channels while the anti-pathogenic factors are not significantly injured. This combination implies an excessive pattern.

Additional notes

1. Is there any evidence of heat in this case?

The patient has yellow urine and a bowel movement only once every two or three days. These two symptoms would generally imply the presence of some heat in the body. However if there is heat, the quantity of urine should be reduced and the stools should be dry, showing that heat has injured the body fluids. This patient has a normal quantity of yellow urine, and although the bowel movement is slow, the stools are moist. The tongue and pulse also show no evidence of heat, thus there is no real indication of heat in this case.

2. Is there evidence of a deficiency pattern?

A thin pulse is generally explained as a reflection of blood and qi deficiency. The pulse appears to be weak because the blood is too scanty to properly fill the vessels. A thin pulse is thus usually a deficiency-type pulse.

However, another indication of a thin pulse is dampness. The pulse can be affected by dampness in two ways. First the dampness blocks the qi and blood circulation. Second the dampness is retained in the tissues which surround the vessels, and this creates pressure which reduces the diameter of the blood vessels. In this case the thin pulse indicates an excessive pattern of disease.

The key to distinguishing whether a thin pulse is deficient or excessive in nature is to be found in the force of the pulse. A thin and forceful pulse implies excess, while a thin and forceless pulse implies deficiency. In this case there was no indication as to whether the pulse was forceful, but all of the other symptoms suggest that there is no deficiency involved.

3. Is there any Kidney deficiency in this case?

Kidney deficiency is a common cause of lower back pain in Chinese medicine. However, it is an interior, not an exterior pattern. This patient has a few symptoms which could possibly indicate that the lower back pain is related to Kidney deficiency: the long history of the disorder, the pulse, and the tongue. However, if the lower back pain were related to Kidney deficiency, the pain would have been continuous and not episodic during its two-year history, and the patient's general condition would be weak.

Conclusion	1. According to the eight principles: Channel-collateral, cold, and excessive pattern. 2. According to etiology: Damp-cold. 3. According to channels and collaterals: Retention of damp-cold in the foot greater yang channel and governing vessel.
Treatment principle	Remove the damp-cold from the channels and collaterals.
Selection of points	GV-3 *(yao yang guan)* B-22 *(san jiao shu)* B-54 *(zhi bian)* Sp-9 *(yin ling quan)*
Explanation of points	GV-3 *(yao yang guan)* effectively removes obstruction from the governing vessel, particularly at the local level. It alleviates pain in the lower back by removing dampness and cold.

B-22 *(san jiao shu)* is the point at which the qi from the Triple Burner channel accumulates. The Triple Burner channel has a strong influence on qi and water metabolism. The presence of dampness and cold restricts the flow of qi, upsetting the normal metabolism of water. Thus, in addition to its local function, this point also has the general function of removing dampness from the body.

B-54 *(zhi bian)* very strongly removes obstruction from the foot greater yang channel. It is effective in treating problems of both the lower back and the lower limbs.

Sp-9 *(yin ling quan)* effectively removes dampness and tonifies the Spleen, especially when the dampness is located in the lower burner.

Combination of points

B-22 *(san jiao shu)* and Sp-9 *(yin ling quan)* are a good combination for treating dampness in the lower burner, the former for regulating the qi in the Triple Burner, and the latter for tonifying the Spleen. They work well together in removing the retention of dampness.

Follow-up

This patient received two treatments on alternate days, after which the lower back pain was much improved and only a feeling of stiffness and cold remained. The appetite was improved and there was no abdominal pain. He was treated five times in the following two weeks after which he had no lower back pain and his appetite was normal. He was advised to wear sensible clothing and to avoid exposure to cold and dampness. There has been no recurrence of the back pain.

CASE 20: **Female, age 42**

Main complaint

Pain in left lower back and lower limb

History

Pain in left lower back and lower limb for ten days with no recent trauma. The patient has a history of recurrent episodes of the same problem. There is also a feeling of coldness, soreness, weakness, numbness and paresthesia over the same area, these symptoms becoming worse when the weather is cold, and the pain becoming more severe. The pain is relieved by warmth and there is no exacerbation of the pain with movement.

There is general lassitude and poor memory, but the patient's appetite is good. She does not sleep soundly and does not feel refreshed on wakening. Bowel movements and urination are normal. The patient has a sallow complexion.

Tongue

Light red body with dry coating, yellow and thick at the root

Pulse

Wiry and forceless

Analysis of symptoms

1. Pain in the lower back and lower limb—
   obstruction of the channels and collaterals.
2. Feeling of coldness and other symptoms become worse in cold weather and are relieved by warmth—retention of pathogenic cold in the channels and collaterals.
3. Soreness, weakness, numbness and paresthesia of the region—
   malnourishment of the channels and collaterals.
4. General lassitude, poor memory, and poor sleep—
   deficiency of qi and blood.
5. Sallow complexion and forceless pulse—deficiency.

Basic theory of case

The channels and collaterals serve as a conduit for the circulation of qi and blood, thus poor circulation caused by a variety of factors will lead to malnourishment of this system, giving rise to different symptoms. Numbness *(má mù)* is a very common clinical symptom. What is called 'numbness' actually consists of two separate problems. The first, *má*, is a subjective alteration of sensation. This corresponds to what is called paresthesia in Western medicine. The second, *mù*, literally 'woodenness,' is a complete loss of sensation and corresponds to what is usually meant by numbness in the West. In this book we will therefore translate *má mù* as numbness and paresthesia.

With paresthesia the patient feels no pain or itching, but an alteration of sensation. Some feel insects crawling on the skin, others complain of a 'pins and needles' sensation, or a very slight electrical stimulation. The symptoms are not relieved by pressure. Paresthesia is usually due to disorders of qi, either stagnation or deficiency.

Numbness is either a complete loss of sensation or reduced sensation. The patient feels that the skin is thick and insensitive, a condition that is not relieved by pressure or movement. When carefully examined, these patients have objective loss of sensation. Numbness usually indicates blood deficiency.

Numbness and paresthesia are often considered to be a single symptom in clinical practice, caused by malnourishment of qi and blood. However, if these problems are the chief complaint, it is important to distinguish between them.

Malnourishment of qi and blood in the channels and collaterals has many different causes, commonly involving qi and blood deficiency or stagnation, or retention of pathogenic factors. In the prodromal or early stage of windstroke the patient may have numbness or paresthesia caused by internal wind; in this type of case the symptom signifies a more serious disorder than it does when caused by other factors.

Fig. 3

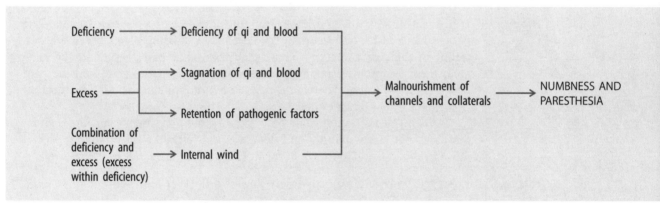

Cause of disease | Pathogenic cold

The patient has symptoms involving pain and coldness of the lower limb which become worse in cold weather and are relieved by warmth. This is characteristic of an invasion by pathogenic cold which 'freezes' or congeals the qi and blood, causing poor circulation and obstruction.

Site of disease | Channels and collaterals

The pain is related to the weather and affects only one side of the body, which means that the site of disease is the body surface, which includes the channels and collaterals.

The patient also has weakness, soreness, numbness, and paresthesia together with general lassitude, poor memory, and poor sleep. This implies that there is qi and blood deficiency internally as well as in the channels and collaterals.

Pathological change | If we compare this to the previous case (number 19) there are some similarities. Both patients experience coldness and pain in the lower back with a preference for warmth. In addition, in both cases the disease is located in the channels and collaterals. But there are also some differences. In this case there is a feeling of coldness and pain in a lower limb, but no heavy sensation, thus the pathogenic factor is cold, but not damp-cold. Here there is also numbness, paresthesia, and weakness of the same region, which suggests deficiency of qi and blood and hence malnourishment of the local tissues, muscles, channels, and collaterals. These symptoms are absent from the previous case.

Malnourishment due to deficiency of qi and blood results in a lowered resistance to invasion by pathogenic factors, and thus a long history of frequent recurrence. In this case there is a mixture of deficiency and excessive patterns, with deficiency of qi and blood and excess of pathogenic cold.

The area in which the patient feels pain involves two channels: the foot greater yang Bladder channel and the foot lesser yang Gallbladder channel. There is also general deficiency of qi and blood which affects the function of the Organs and causes general lassitude, poor memory, and poor sleep. Because the face is deprived of nourishment the patient's complexion is sallow, yet the normal red coloration of the tongue body suggests that the qi and blood deficiency is not severe. The wiry pulse indicates pain and also the involvement of the lesser yang channel, yet it is forceless because of the deficiency.

Fig. 4

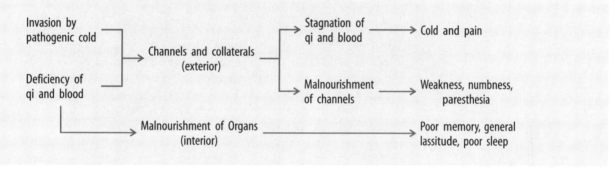

| Pattern of disease | The retention of pathogenic cold in the channels and collaterals indicates a channel-collateral pattern. The deficiency of qi and blood indicates that there is also an interior pattern. |

The retention of pathogenic cold in the channels and collaterals indicates a channel-collateral pattern. The deficiency of qi and blood indicates that there is also an interior pattern.

The feeling of coldness and pain on the lower limb and the patient's preference for warmth indicates a cold pattern.

There are symptoms of deficiency both internally and in the channels, but there is also retention of pathogenic cold in the channels; the pattern is thus both deficient and excessive.

Additional notes

1. Is there dysfunction of the Heart or Spleen in this case?

The Heart governs the blood and the Spleen is the source of qi and blood. The main symptoms of Heart blood deficiency are palpitations and insomnia, whereas Spleen qi deficiency is characterized by poor appetite and digestive problems. The poor sleep in this case is trivial compared to typical insomnia and is of minor importance here. The patient has a good appetite, and the poor memory and general lassitude cannot be connected to any particular Organ. The diagnosis can therefore only be one of general qi and blood deficiency, rather than a problem specifically involving the Heart or Spleen.

2. Is there any Kidney disorder?

Soreness and weakness of the lower back and knee joints is one of the main symptoms of a Kidney disorder. In this case, however, the symptoms occur only on one side. There is also pain and numbness and paresthesia caused by retention of cold and deficiency of qi and blood in the channels. There is no evidence of Kidney deficiency.

3. What is the cause of numbness and paresthesia in this case?

Numbness and paresthesia can be caused by either deficiency or excess. In cases where a mixture of excess and deficiency exists, it is always necessary to determine which aspect is primary. Here, although both aspects are present, the deficiency of qi and blood in the channels is the primary cause of the disorder. There is a long history of general qi and blood deficiency, and the pain is not really severe. (Pain, numbness, and paresthesia caused by cold tends to be very severe in character.)

4. Why does the patient have a dry, yellow, and thick coating on the root of the tongue?

The root of the tongue reflects the condition of the lower burner and the lower part of the Stomach. The thick coating indicates an interior problem, and the dry coating (which is also yellow) indicates heat. Generally speaking, all of these signs mean that there is retention of heat in the Stomach and lower burner.

When there is a single sign or symptom which does not fit into the general pattern of a case, we suggest the following method to assess its significance. First, examine the history to find any evidence that would support the aberrant finding. In this case one would look for evidence supporting the presence of heat. There may be phlegm, retention of food, or heat in the Large Intestine or Bladder. If even one symptom could be found, the diagnosis would have to change to one in which there is a mixture of heat and cold. In this case the patient has a good appetite and normal urination and bowel movements. None of these findings supports a diagnosis of heat. Second, look for some extraneous reason for the aberrant finding. In patients with tongues that do not match your diagnosis be sure to check for other factors which could affect the tongue, such as recent activity, medicine, food, or smoking. If any of these factors are present you can disregard the coating. If not you must conclude that the symptom is simply false. It is essential to determine which symptoms are true and which are false and can thus be ignored.

In this case all the symptoms indicate a pattern of cold, the tongue coating alone being contradictory; it can thus be disregarded.

Conclusion

1. According to the eight principles diagnosis:
   This pattern is channel-collateral and interior, cold, and both deficient and excessive. The deficiency is at the level of qi and blood, the excess in the channel.

2. According to etiology diagnosis:
   Pathogenic cold.

3. According to channels and collaterals diagnosis:
   Retention of cold in the foot greater yang and lesser yang channels.

4. According to qi and blood diagnosis:
   Qi and blood deficiency.

Treatment principle

Remove the pathogenic cold and obstruction from the channels and alleviate the pain.

Selection of points

B-36 *(cheng fu)*
B-40 *(wei zhong)*
G-31 *(feng shi)*
G-40 *(qiu xu)*
hua tuo jia ji (M-BW-35) on the left at the level of T11 and L3
B-20 *(pi shu)*
B-24 *(qi hai shu)*
Ashi point

Two *hua tuo jia ji* (M-BW-35) points and two points on the Bladder channel were selected on the side with the problem, two above and two below the main area of tenderness or pain. *See Fig. 5.*

Fig. 5

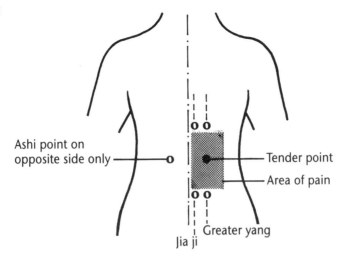

Ashi point on opposite side only — o

Tender point

Area of pain

Greater yang

Jia ji

Explanation of points

B-36 *(cheng fu)* and B-40 *(wei zhong)* remove obstruction from the Bladder channel.

G-31 *(feng shi)* and G-40 *(qiu xu)* remove obstruction from the Gallbladder channel.

These two pairs of points promote the circulation of qi and blood in the two involved channels, and also help relieve the lower back pain. Warm needle technique can be used at these points.

The *hua tuo jia ji (M-BW-35)* and local Bladder channel points were used to accomplish the same goal locally.

In this case it is important to avoid using too many points, since the use of too many needles could further injure the qi.

Follow-up

After one treatment the lower back pain was gone, but the patient still felt weakness and soreness in the lower limbs. Her general symptoms did not change, so the point prescription was modified to address the problem of general qi and blood deficiency. The new prescription was as follows:

B-20 *(pi shu)*
B-23 *(shen shu)*
B-36 *(cheng fu)*
B-40 *(wei zhong)*
G-31 *(feng shi)*

The patient was treated twice a week for two weeks, after which her energy level was much improved and her legs no longer felt weak.

CASE 21: **Male, age 67**

Main complaint

Soreness in the lower back

History

Four days ago the patient developed a slight fever and an aversion to cold; the symptoms are still present. The patient has distention in the epigastrium and abdomen, and also complains of nausea and a complete loss of appetite. There is excessive saliva in the mouth accompanied by a diminished sense of taste. There is pain and soreness of the back, especially in the lumbar area, and the patient also complains of a sensation of heaviness and restriction of movement in the lower back. The head, spinal column, shoulders, and knee joints all feel heavy and restricted, but to a lesser degree.

Tongue	Slightly dark red body, thin, moist, and slightly yellow coating
Pulse	Slippery and slightly floating, thin on the left side proximal position

Analysis of symptoms

1. Aversion to cold and slight fever—
   retention of pathogenic factors in the superficial tissues.
2. Soreness and heaviness in the lower back, shoulders, and back—
   pathogenic dampness in the channels and collaterals.
3. Nausea, upper and middle abdominal distention, anorexia with diminished
   sensation of taste—retention of dampness in the Stomach and Spleen.
4. Thin and moist tongue coating, slippery and slightly floating pulse—
   retention of pathogenic dampness in the superficial tissues.

Basic theory of case

When external pathogenic factors attack the body they generally reside in the superficial tissues where they establish an exterior pattern of disease. If they are not expelled but remain in the body for a long period of time, they can migrate inwards to the Organs and establish an interior pattern.

During this transformation from exterior to interior there may be symptoms of both an exterior and interior pattern. In other cases, however, the pathogenic factors go immediately from the exterior to the interior without displaying any mixed, transitional symptoms. This is more likely to be the case, e.g., when wind-cold or wind-heat attack the body surface and manifest as exterior cold or heat patterns. If these pathogens are retained they can give rise to an interior heat pattern.

By contrast, during the onset of an attack by pathogenic dampness there is usually a combination of interior and exterior patterns. The site of the interior pattern is in the Spleen and Stomach because of the association of the Spleen with the body's water metabolism. When dampness invades it is retained in the body, disrupting the function of the Spleen; this explains why the patient shows symptoms of both external dampness and retention of internal dampness.

Fig. 6

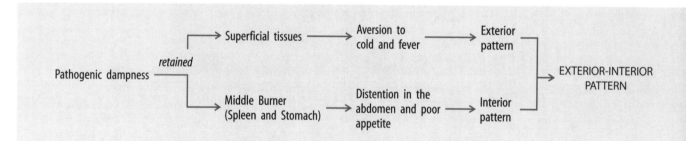

Cause of disease

Pathogenic dampness

The patient has soreness and a feeling of heaviness in many areas of the body, together with abdominal distention, nausea, and anorexia. These are evidence of turbid dampness. The patient has only a four-day history of illness, starting with an aversion to cold and a temperature. These symptoms suggest that the patient was attacked by pathogenic dampness from the environment.

Site of disease

1. Superficial tissues
2. Stomach and Spleen

The main evidence suggesting that the patient's disease is located in the superficial tissues includes aversion to cold accompanied by a slight fever; soreness, heaviness, and pain in the lower back, knees, upper back, spinal column, head, and shoulders; and the floating pulse.

The main evidence suggesting that the Stomach and Spleen are the site of the disease includes the nausea, anorexia, loss of taste, epigastric and abdominal distention.

Pathological change

This case exhibits a combination of interior and exterior patterns. The cause of the condition was an invasion of pathogenic factors. The manifestations can be divided into three different layers: the superficial tissues, the channels and collaterals, and the Organs.

There is no clear history of exposure to pathogenic factors in this case, but the patient does have a fever and aversion to cold which implies retention of pathogenic factors within the superficial tissues, leading to stagnation of the protective qi. Thus we know that the condition was caused by external factors.

The patient has very obvious symptoms of pain and discomfort in many areas of the body. The characteristic of the pain is that it affects large areas; moreover, it is accompanied by both soreness and heaviness. That large areas are affected indicates involvement of the channels and collaterals. Pathogenic factors pervade the atmosphere and envelop the body, making invasion of widespread areas of the body surface possible. This results in very extensive obstruction of qi and blood within the superficial tissues. The patient especially complained of soreness and heaviness in the lower back, thus we can infer that the foot greater yang Bladder channel and governing vessel are most seriously obstructed. The soreness and heaviness signify an invasion of dampness.

The loss of appetite and abdominal distention are symptoms of abnormal digestive function. The middle burner functions of transportation and transformation are impaired, as dampness has seriously obstructed the flow of qi in this area. As a result the clear qi cannot ascend and the turbid qi cannot descend; it is this stagnation in the middle burner that causes distention of the abdomen. The turbid qi reverses its directional flow and rises up, leading to nausea. Food therefore cannot be digested properly and is retained; this weakens the Stomach's ability to accept food, causing anorexia.

The Spleen opens through the mouth and controls the sense of taste; a disorder of the Stomach and Spleen may thus lead to irregularities in the sense of taste. For example, sweet, sour, and rancid tastes, as well as sticky or greasy sensations in the mouth, may occur as a result of Spleen dysfunction. In this case the patient's ability to taste food is diminished. Tastelessness is a very common symptom, and the cause is often invasion of the Spleen by pathogenic dampness, as occurred here.

The combination of exterior and interior disease patterns may occur under two sets of circumstances. In the first, the interior and exterior patterns may be caused by the same pathogenic factor, and hence the two patterns are related to each other. In the second, the interior and exterior disorders have different causes, e.g., a patient with a pre-existing interior pattern is later attacked by external pathogenic factors; the interior and exterior patterns are thus independent of one another. In this case there are three different sites of disease, but the cause is the same, i.e., external dampness. The fact that the symptoms occurred simultaneously is a strong indication of a single cause of disease. *See Fig. 7.*

The moist tongue coating and slippery pulse are a result of pathogenic dampness. The tongue coating is still thin, and the pulse is slightly floating, because the patient has not fully recovered from the exterior pattern.

Pattern of disease

The dampness is retained in the superficial tissues and in the Spleen and Stomach, thus this is a combination of interior and exterior patterns.

The pronounced aversion to cold, slight fever without thirst, and tastelessness suggest a cold pattern.

The retention of dampness and obstruction of qi indicate an excessive pattern.

Fig. 7

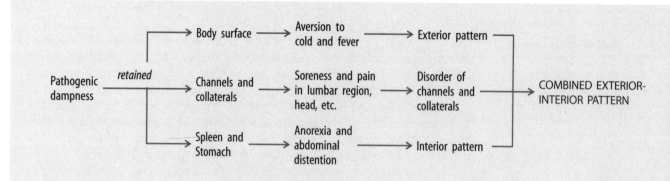

Additional notes

1. Is there enough evidence of heat in this patient's symptoms to constitute a heat pattern?

The patient has a slightly dark red tongue with a hint of yellow on the coating, signs which are characteristic of heat. These symptoms are present because of the retention of dampness in the middle burner, causing the yang qi to stagnate and transform into heat. From analysis of this patient's case, it is clear that there are no obvious heat symptoms, but merely a potential for a heat pattern to develop. These few symptoms do not yet constitute a heat pattern for purposes of diagnosis.

Case number 20 involved only a channel disorder, and the singular presence of cold. In this case, however, there are problems in both the channels and the interior (involving the Organs). Consequently there is a greater tendency for the pattern to transform into one of heat.

The yang qi of the body circulates from the inside to the outside and is therefore much stronger within the Organs than in the superficial tissues. When pathogenic dampness invades the body, obstruction of the yang qi can occur. In case number 20 the stagnation was confined to the superficial tissues and channels; in this case the obstruction is in the channels and collaterals, but also in the middle burner. This leads to a greater tendency towards heat.

2. Does the patient have Kidney deficiency?

The health of the Kidney is reflected in the pulse at the proximal position, and in this case the quality of the pulse is thin at this position only. There is thus deficiency of the Kidney. However, based on our analysis of the symptoms it is clear that pathogenic dampness is the main cause of disease, and although Kidney deficiency is present, it is not severe. The patient has a very short history of illness, and it is thus impossible to diagnose as a pattern of Kidney deficiency. Moreover, the thin pulse cannot be regarded as a symptom of dampness in this case because it is only present in one of the three pulse positions.

3. Does the patient have Spleen qi deficiency?

Both retention of dampness in the middle burner and Spleen qi deficiency can cause abnormal digestion, but the symptoms are different; moreover, one is an excessive pattern and the other is deficient. The pattern in this case is one of excess, and there is no deficiency of Spleen qi. This distinction was explained earlier in the section on pathological change.

Conclusion

1. According to the eight principles diagnosis:
   Exterior and interior, cold, and excessive.
2. According to etiology:
   External pathogenic dampness.

3. According to channels and collaterals:
   Retention of dampness, mainly in the foot greater yang Bladder channel and governing vessel.
4. According to Organ theory:
   Retention of dampness in the Spleen and Stomach.

Treatment principle

1. Remove dampness and obstruction from the channels and collaterals.
2. Resolve dampness and regulate the qi of the middle burner.

Selection of the points

GV-14 *(da zhui)*
GV-8 *(jin suo)*
Sp-9 *(yin ling quan)*
Two sets of Ashi points: near B-15 *(xin shu)* and slightly lateral to B-23 *(shen shu)*

Explanation of points

GV-14 *(da zhui)* is the meeting point of the seven yang channels, and regulates the qi in the yang channels. It also helps expel external pathogenic factors. In this case it is used to help remove the dampness from the channels. And because the patient complains of discomfort in the upper back, it is also used for its local effects.

GV-8 *(jin suo)* is located below the spinous process of the ninth thoracic vertebra. This is quite close to the level of the middle burner, and the point is thus a good choice for regulating the Stomach and Spleen qi. By improving the qi function, it helps resolve the retention of dampness. The point is also effective in strengthening the spinal column, particularly when there is stiffness, pain, and spasm on or around the spine.

Sp-9 *(yin ling quan)* regulates and tonifies the Spleen qi. It is especially useful for removing dampness from the body. As it is close to the knee joints, it is also used for its local effects.

The Ashi points help alleviate pain by relieving the local obstruction. They are chosen primarily to help with the main complaint.

Follow-up

This patient was treated daily for two days, after which the bad cold and the soreness and heaviness around the body were resolved. However, he still complained of discomfort in the lower back and poor appetite. The point prescription was therefore modified to tonify the Spleen and remove dampness:

P-6 *(nei guan)*
B-17 *(ge shu)*
B-20 *(pi shu)*
Sp-9 *(yin ling quan)*
Ashi point on the lower back

He was treated daily for five days with the new prescription, after which he made a complete recovery.

CASE 22: **Male, age 41**

Main complaint

Lower back pain

History

This patient overexerted himself at work. After lifting a heavy object he developed severe pain in the lower back. At the time movement in the lower back was unaffected, but the following morning the pain was very severe and his movement was severely restricted. Every movement caused sharp pain, making it difficult for the patient to walk. The pain radiated downwards over the buttocks and both legs. Besides the pain the patient did not feel any other discomfort. He received several *tui na* treatments without effective relief, and came for acupuncture the third morning after the injury. His general health is good.

The tongue and pulse are normal.

Analysis of symptoms

1. Lower back pain—obstruction of the channels and collaterals.
2. History of trauma and severe pain—blood stasis.

Basic theory of case

In Chinese medicine, trauma is considered a frequent cause of disease. Trauma usually results from improper physical activity or accidents at the work place. The primary manifestations are hemorrhage (including subcutaneous bleeding and bruising), swelling, and pain. These characteristics are only applicable to accidents which do not involve fractures or direct injury of the viscera.

The symptoms of local trauma mainly involve the skin, channels and collaterals, and muscles, although under certain conditions the sinews and vessels may also be involved. The impact of the trauma directly influences the local area, and often this restricts the flow of blood, resulting in blood stasis. Even when there is hemorrhage, blood stasis may develop at a later stage.

Cause of disease

Trauma

The patient has a history of trauma which occurred at work. The main symptom is severe pain in the lower back, and this implies an injury of the channels and collaterals. This patient's history and symptoms are very clear, and thus the cause of disease in this case is trauma.

Site of disease

Channels and collaterals

The history and symptoms clearly reveal the site of the disease; moreover this patient's general health is very good. He has no other abnormal symptoms, thus the Organs are not involved in this case.

Pathological change

The local channels and muscles of the lower back were injured by overexertion. The circulation of blood was thereby retarded, which led to blood stasis, which in turn increased the obstruction in the channel and thus the pain.

Initially there was only a channel and collateral, muscle injury, and the pain was not too severe. Blood stasis then developed, the pain intensified, and restriction of movement resulted. This is why the patient's pain evolved from severe to very severe.

Although the pain is very severe the trauma has only caused local injury to the channels and collaterals. The injury has not affected the general function of qi, blood, or the Organs. This explains why the patient has no other symptoms involving his general condition, and why the complexion, tongue, and pulse reflect no abnormality.

Pattern of disease

Because trauma caused the injury to the channel and collateral, this is a channel-collateral pattern. The Organs are not affected.

There is no cold or heat manifestation.

Blood stasis in the channels and collaterals is an excessive pattern.

Additional notes

The trauma patient has a clear and short history of illness. In the clinical situation this makes it very easy to diagnose the disorder.

The ability to recognize blood stasis is very important. The characteristic symptom is the presence of sharp and stabbing pain. In reality, however, very few acute trauma patients exhibit this symptom. Furthermore, the tongue and pulse cannot be relied upon in acute disorders. The accuracy of these indicators in acute disorders is dependent on two factors: the extent of the blood stasis, and whether there has been enough time since onset for change to occur.

Diagnosis of blood stasis in trauma is not only based on the symptoms. The history of the illness and the analysis of the pathological change is even more important. Regardless of how severe or slight the trauma, blood stasis will sooner or later be the result.

Some patients develop chronic lower back pain as a result of an old injury. The symptoms at onset may have been severe or slight, but the principle of diagnosis for this type of patient is the same as for the acute type. Blood stasis is still regarded as the main problem. There are two possible causes of blood stasis in chronic cases. The first is when the stagnation occurred long before and was never completely healed. The second is when the patient has a history of very slight injury to the channel and collateral, and the injury is so slight that it takes a long time for stagnation to develop.

The chronic lower back pain patient usually has a host of accompanying symptoms. The dysfunction can manifest in one of the Organs or on a general qi and blood level, and when this occurs it is categorized as a combination of channel-collateral and interior pattern.

Conclusion

1. According to the eight principles:
   Channel-collateral pattern, absence of heat or cold, excessive pattern.

2. According to etiology:
   Trauma.

3. According to channels and collaterals:
   Stagnation of the qi and blood in the foot greater yang channels.

4. According to qi, blood, and body fluids:
   Blood stasis and qi stagnation.

Treatment principle

1. Remove the obstruction from the channels and collaterals.
2. Alleviate the pain.

Point selection

B-63 *(jin men)*

Explanation of point

B-63 *(jin men)* is the accumulating point of the foot greater yang Bladder channel. It works very effectively to remove obstruction from the qi and blood levels in the channel.

Follow-up

The pain disappeared instantly and did not recur.

Diagnostic principles for lower back pain

Lower back pain is one of the most common problems encountered in the practice of acupuncture. The diagnosis rests mainly on the cause and also the pathological change.

1. Cause of disease

There are three main causes of lower back pain: invasion by pathogenic factors, Kidney deficiency, and trauma.

a) Invasion by pathogenic factors

The most common pathogenic factor is dampness, particularly cold and dampness together. Sometimes the invasion may be due to damp-heat, but this is much less common. The pathogenic factors that influence the body are in the environment, but are different from those which cause exterior patterns.

In the case of exterior patterns, the common pathogenic factors are wind-cold and wind-heat, dampness being involved less frequently. The whole body is affected and the symptoms are generalized in nature, just as wind, heat, and cold are present throughout the environment.

Dampness, on the other hand, tends to be heavy and low-lying. Patients are often affected by dampness if they live in cold and damp areas, have poor housing, or work underground or in cold and damp conditions. The lower back and lower limbs are usually affected because the dampness comes from the ground, and also because when it invades the body the symptoms tend to be localized in the lower part of the body.

Fig. 8

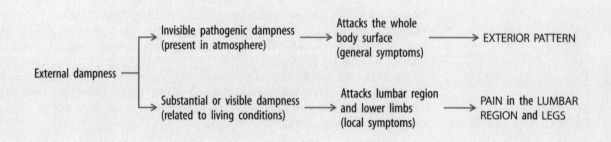

b) Kidney deficiency

In basic Chinese theory the lower back is described as the 'dwelling of the Kidney', thus the Kidney supports and nourishes this region. Kidney deficiency patterns almost always involve lower back pain, whether it is the main symptom or merely a minor part of a Kidney deficiency disorder.

Fig. 9

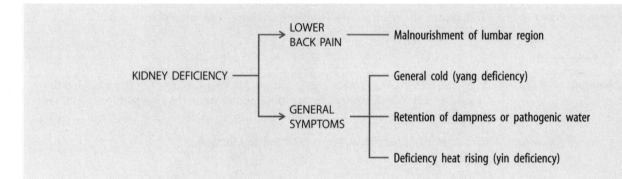

c) Trauma

Chronic lower back pain can be caused by bad posture over a long period of time while doing physical labor.

In acute cases there is usually a clear history of having fallen, lifted a heavy object, or suffered local injury from direct violence to the back. Sometimes the patient cannot identify an obvious cause of the trauma, but the symptoms suggest this rather than invasion by pathogenic factors.

2. Pathological change

When dampness invades the lower back it causes obstruction of qi in the channels and collaterals, leading to localized pain. Kidney deficiency is an internal cause of lower back pain which results in malnourishment of the structures in the local area. The patient will complain of weakness and dull pain.

Trauma influences the channels, collaterals, muscles, vessels, and even the bone, thus the injury is at both the qi and blood levels, which is the case from the time that the injury is sustained. Blood stasis can also occur when there is invasion by dampness, but only after a considerable period of time.

Fig. 10

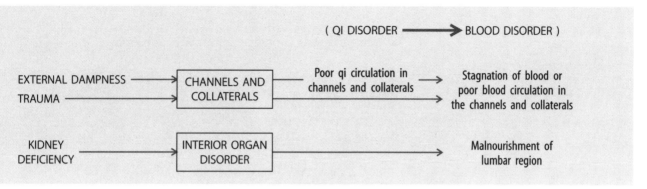

3. Key points in the diagnosis of lower back pain

There are two main considerations: the characteristics of the lower back pain itself, and the accompanying symptoms.

a) Lower back pain caused by dampness

The lower back pain may be mild or severe and is frequently accompanied by a local sensation of heaviness. The pain is closely related to changes in the weather. If the lower back pain is caused by damp-cold the patient will have a cold feeling in the lower back, and the pain is aggravated upon exposure to cold. There is no fever, and the patient will not be thirsty. The urine may be copious and pale in color, and the stools are moist. The tongue coating is white and greasy, and the pulse may vary in quality but is never rapid.

When the lower back pain is caused by damp-heat there will be a local feeling of heat in the lower back, and there may be fever. The urine is yellow and there is dysuria and even hematuria. The stools are dry. The tongue is red with a yellow, greasy coating and the pulse is rapid.

In the clinical situation lower back pain due to damp-cold is much more common than that due to damp-heat. Some patients can recall an episode of working or living in damp, low-lying areas.

b) Lower back pain caused by Kidney deficiency

The pain is not very severe; rather the patient complains of a dull pain, and the history is usually prolonged. There is no obvious relationship to changes in the weather, and the patient gives no history of exposure to pathogenic factors. In addition to lower back pain, the patient will complain of soreness and weakness of the lower back and possibly the knees, and he may have difficulty in standing for any period of time. Sometimes the patient will support the lower back with his hands, as this tends to relieve the feeling of soreness and weakness.

In the case of Kidney yang deficiency there will also be symptoms such as feeling cold, with cold extremities, edema, diarrhea, and copious, clear urine.

If there is Kidney yin deficiency the patient will have afternoon fevers, night sweats, or heat in the five centers. The urine will be yellow and the stools dry.

c) Lower back pain caused by trauma

This type of patient has the most severe pain, with a short history involving injury. The pain may be the only symptom. There may well be no other symptoms, thus the diagnosis is straightforward.

d) Chronic lower back pain

These patients have a very long history in which qi stagnation has eventually led to blood stasis. The initial cause of the lower back pain varies, but after such a long period the symptoms have changed and are now those of blood stasis in the channel. In the clinical situation it may be difficult to precisely classify this type of backache.

Fig. 11   4. The entire diagnostic procedure for lower back pain is summarized in Figure 11.

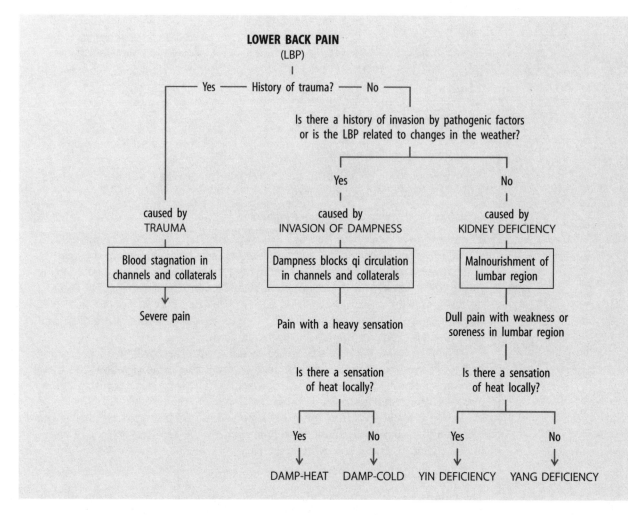

Painful Obstruction
(Bi Syndrome)

CASE 23: **Female, age 41**

Main complaint

Joint pain in the fingers, wrists, and elbows

History

This woman worked as a cleaner in a small factory for over ten years where she had contact with cold water. Two months ago she began to get pains in all the small joints of her fingers, particularly severe at the finger tips. The pain worsens in cold weather and towards the end of each working day, but eases in warm surroundings. When the pain is aggravated, it radiates from the fingers to the wrists and elbows. Recently the pain in the wrists and elbows has become as bad as that in the fingers.

She also complains of poor sleep, palpitations, and a stifling sensation in the chest. Her appetite, bowels, and urination are normal. Her finger nails have recently become flatter than usual and have lost their luster. Her energy level is poor, especially during menstruation, but the period is otherwise normal. Sometimes she feels a slight soreness and weakness in the lower back, and the knee joints have a mildly uncomfortable feeling when she walks, especially when descending stairs.

Tongue

Slightly pale body, two areas of ecchymosis (middle and right side), coating is thin and white

Pulse

Sunken and moderate

Analysis of symptoms

1. Contact with cold water for prolonged period—
   invasion by pathogenic damp-cold.
2. Cold pain in the joints which worsens with exposure to cold and improves with warmth—obstruction of the channels.
3. Soreness and weakness of the lower back, uncomfortable knees—
   poor circulation of qi and blood.
4. Stifling sensation in the chest—stagnation of qi.
5. Palpitations and poor sleep—malnourishment of the spirit.

6. Ecchymosis on the tongue—blood stasis.

7. Sunken and moderate pulse—obstruction of the channels by damp-cold.

Basic theory of case

Painful obstruction *(bì zhèng)* is a traditional Chinese disease classification dating back to the *Inner Classic*. In fact, one entire chapter of *Basic Questions* is devoted to this subject. In a general sense, the term refers to obstruction of qi and blood by pathogenic factors. In a more narrow context, however, it refers to external pathogenic factors which only locally obstruct the channels and thereby affect the joints, bones, sinews, and soft tissues. This can lead to joint disorders with soreness, pain, swelling, numbness, paresthesia, limitation of movement, and deformity. In a clinical situation both aspects of the term painful obstruction are utilized, but the narrow meaning is more commonly used.

Because the general type of painful obstruction refers to disorders on many different levels throughout the body, the general pattern is further differentiated into two broad categories, the first based upon the depth of tissue affected, the second upon penetration of the yin Organs.

1. Depth of tissue affected

i.   Skin painful obstruction: the pathogenic factors are obstructing the superficial level of the body. The symptom common to this pattern is reduced or lost sensation.

ii. Muscle painful obstruction: the pathogenic factors have penetrated to the muscular layer. The symptoms are soreness, muscle aches, stiffness, and deeper numbness or paresthesia.

iii. Vessel painful obstruction: the pathogenic factors have reached the vessels. At this stage the disease is changing from a qi level to a blood level disorder. There will be purplish dark areas and the pain will be of the cold type. In severe cases gangrene can set in. There may be aching pain along the whole channel.

iv. Sinew painful obstruction: at this stage the pathogenic factors are penetrating to a very deep layer. The symptoms are inflexibility with stiffness, spasms, or pain.

v.   Bone painful obstruction: this is the deepest layer of penetration. The primary manifestations are bone weakness and deformity.

2. Yin Organs. The second category of general painful obstruction is that in which the yin Organs are affected. They are variously called Heart painful obstruction, Lung painful obstruction, Spleen painful obstruction, Liver painful obstruction, and Kidney painful obstruction. Details of their presentations will be analyzed in the cases in this chapter. *See Fig. 1.*

Cause of disease

Damp-cold

The patient has a long history of regular contact with cold water and the characteristics are cold pain in the affected areas with a desire for warmth. These symptoms show that it is a pure yin pathogenic factor which attacks the yang qi of the body. Damp-cold is the cause of the disorder, with cold predominating.

Site of disease

Joints

The primary symptoms occur in the elbow, wrist, and finger joints.

Pathological change

The basic pathological change is that the external pathogenic factors are obstructing the circulation of qi and blood, which causes joint pain. While there are many possible combinations of pathogenic factors that can bring about painful obstruction, in this case they are cold and dampness. The patient's ten year contact with water is the obvious cause of the damp-cold. When the antipathogenic factor is

Fig. 1

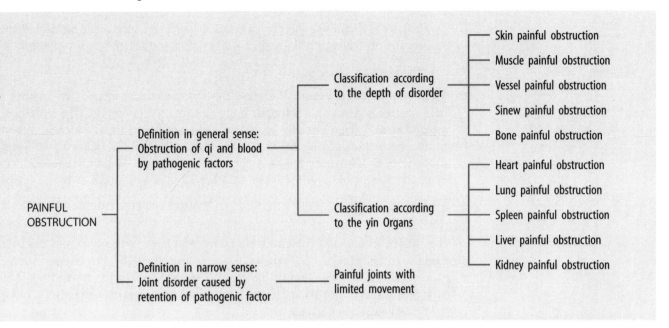

PAINFUL OBSTRUCTION

Definition in general sense: Obstruction of qi and blood by pathogenic factors

Classification according to the depth of disorder
- Skin painful obstruction
- Muscle painful obstruction
- Vessel painful obstruction
- Sinew painful obstruction
- Bone painful obstruction

Classification according to the yin Organs
- Heart painful obstruction
- Lung painful obstruction
- Spleen painful obstruction
- Liver painful obstruction
- Kidney painful obstruction

Definition in narrow sense: Joint disorder caused by retention of pathogenic factor

Painful joints with limited movement

strong the disorder will not emerge, but prolonged exposure to pathogenic cold and dampness can eventually weaken the antipathogenic factor and hence the local yang qi. This process would have been assisted by the slow but gradual decline in the patient's resistance caused by aging. In Chinese medicine the four limbs are regarded as the extremities of yang. This implies that the yang in the limbs is weaker than that within the trunk. When the pathogenic factors attacked, the symptoms began at the weakest point of yang, i.e., the extremities of the limbs.

Pathogenic cold is characterized by constriction and stagnation. It blocks the circulation of qi and blood in the channels, causing pain. Any additional exposure to cold will aggravate the stagnation and intensify the pain. Warmth will improve the circulation and reduce the pain.

Menstruation is a normal process which involves the loss of blood. Short-term mild lassitude is not unusual before or during the period because the qi pushes the blood down, preparing it for discharge. In this case the patient's yang qi is deficient as a result of the long-term exposure to cold. This is aggravated by the further loss of qi during menstruation, bringing about more fatigue or lassitude.

The lower back supports most of the weight of the body. When the yang qi is injured, soreness and weakness may emerge. The patient's posture during work will contribute to these mild symptoms.

This woman also has more long-term complaints, such as a stifling sensation in the chest, palpitations, and poor sleep. They are mainly caused by qi deficiency and the consequent poor circulation of blood in the upper burner. Her sleep has been impaired because the spirit has been deprived of its normal nourishment; yet no heat is present and thus her sleep in not disturbed by dreams.

The slightly pale tongue and white coating indicate retention of cold. The ecchymosis indicates poor blood circulation. The sunken and moderate pulse indicates the presence of damp-cold in the channels and stagnation of qi and blood.

Pattern of disease   Channel-collateral pattern combined with interior yang qi deficiency. The pathogenic damp-cold has attacked the joints but has not influenced the sinews and bones. Therefore only the channels are affected. The long-term exposure to cold has brought about yang qi deficiency.

In this case the pathogenic factor is obviously damp-cold. There is no evidence of heat.

This case is a combination of excess and deficiency. Excess is the main problem because the obstruction of qi and blood is the reason for the pain in the joints.

Additional notes

1. Is there blood stasis in this case?

When we analyzed the cause of disease only damp-cold was mentioned. However, there was ecchymosis on the tongue body and this commonly signifies that there is blood stasis. There actually is some evidence of blood stasis which is caused by the obstruction of the channels from damp-cold and the injury to the yang qi of the body. However, this was not mentioned in the diagnosis because it is secondary damp-cold and there are no other signs or symptoms of blood stasis.

2. What is the relationship between the channel-collateral pattern and interior disorder?

The channel-collateral problem is the main complaint in this case and the first objective of treatment is to eliminate it. The patient also suffers from palpitations, poor sleep, stifling sensation in the chest, and weakness of the lower back, but these symptoms are not severe. If the channel problem is treated correctly the other problems will gradually improve.

The patient has a long history of exposure to cold, yet the channel disorder only emerged two months ago. This fact, combined with the patient's relatively young age, implies that her general resistance is still fairly good. When the pathogenic factors are expelled from the channel, the antipathogenic factor will recover and the yang qi of the entire body will improve.

3. What caused the patient's nail problem?

In Chinese medicine the nails are an extension of the sinews. There is a famous saying which states that "The nails are the surplus of the sinews." The Liver also manifests in the nails. This patient has flat and lusterless nails, palpitations, and a pale tongue, which could be diagnosed as blood or Liver blood deficiency. However, in this case there is no other evidence that would support either diagnosis.

There is poor circulation of blood, but it is due to the invasion of pathogenic factors. This local problem is why the nails are malnourished.

Fig. 2

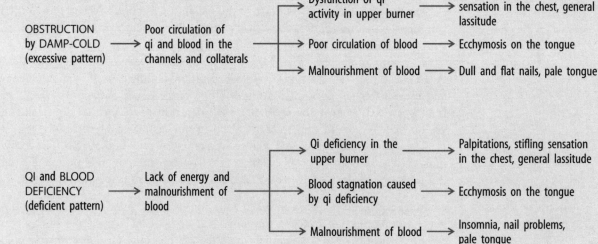

Conclusion

1. According to the eight principles:
   Combination of channel-collateral and interior, cold, and both excess and deficiency patterns. Excess is the main problem.

2. According to etiology:
   Invasion of damp-cold.

3. According to channels and collaterals:
   Obstruction of the channels by damp-cold.

4. According to yin-yang theory:
   Deficiency of yang qi.

Treatment principle

1. Remove the damp-cold.
2. Relieve the obstruction in the channels.
3. Alleviate the pain.
4. Assist the yang qi.

Selection of points

TB-5 *(wai guan)*
SI-6 *(yang lao)* with warm needle. These two points were needled alternately.
ba xie (M-UE-22)
TB-10 *(tian jing)*
S-36 *(zu san li)*
xi yan (M-LE-16)

Explanation of points

TB-5 *(wai guan)* removes obstruction from the channel and alleviates pain. It is the meeting point of the yang linking vessel, and is therefore particularly effective in expelling external pathogenic factors. It also has the local effect of relieving pain in nearby joints. By puncturing this point deeply, P-6 *(nei guan)* will be stimulated to treat the chest symptoms.

SI-6 *(yang lao)* is the accumulating point of the hand greater yang channel. This point relaxes the sinews, alleviates pain, and clears obstruction from the channel. *Yăng lăo* means 'nourishing the old' in Chinese. It is often punctured in the aged for chronic lower back pain. This patient has soreness in the lower back and injury to the yang qi, thus the point is used alternately with TB-5 *(wai guan)* to treat the cold both in its superficial and deep aspects.

ba xie (M-UE-22) reduce swelling and alleviate pain in the fingers and hand. These points also remove local obstruction from the channels.

TB-10 *(tian jing)* removes pathogenic factors and obstruction from the hand lesser yang channel. It also helps to alleviate the local elbow pain.

S-36 *(zu san li)* removes obstruction from the yang brightness channel, alleviates the local knee pain, and promotes the antipathogenic factor.

xi yan (M-LE-16) promotes the local circulation of qi and blood.

Combination of points

S-36 *(zu san li)* and TB-5 *(wai guan)*: Both points are chosen from the channels with the greatest quantity of yang qi. S-36 *(zu san li)* is on the yang brightness channel, which is richest in qi and blood, and TB-5 *(wai guan)* is on the Triple Burner channel, which controls the source qi. The use of S-36 *(zu san li)* supports the internal aspects of the body by promoting qi and yang, while TB-5 *(wai guan)* which is connected with the yang linking vessel promotes the protective qi in the superficial aspects of the body. By thus using TB-5 *(wai guan)* and S-36 *(zu san li)* the proper functioning of the body is promoted both in its interior and exterior aspects.

xi yan (M-LE-16) and S-36 *(zu san li)*: This pair is the most commonly utilized combination in the clinic for knee joint pain. *Xi yan* is located in the small cavities on either side of the knee through which the pathogenic factors often get into the knee joint. By puncturing these points they can be driven out. S-36 *(zu san li)* has a powerful local effect as well as a broader ability to promote the general resistance of the body. This pair of points can thereby be used for either deficient or excessive conditions.

Follow-up

The patient received treatment three times per week. After one week the finger pain was much improved and the cold symptoms were nearly gone. After the second week of treatment all the symptoms had disappeared. She was advised to change her job and to take the following Chinese herbs for one week:

Ramulus Cinnamomi Cassiae *(gui zhi)*   Rhizoma Zingiberis Officinalis Recens *(sheng jiang)*
Radix Paeoniae Lactiflorae *(bai shao)*   Radix Lateralis Aconiti Carmichaeli Praeparata *(fu zi)*
Ramulus Mori Albae *(sang zhi)*   Radix Glycyrrhizae Uralensis *(gan cao)*

Her hands were still a little bit cold but not painful during the first winter after treatment. She kept her hands warm and required no further treatment.

CASE 24: **Male, age 28**

Main complaint

Joint pain

History

The patient has a history of rheumatoid arthritis with episodes of pain and swelling of joints. This disease began six years ago with symptoms primarily of the knees and ankles, but also occasionally involving his elbows and wrists.

One week ago he developed a bad cold with aversion to cold, fever, and a sore throat. Three days ago his left knee and ankle joints became swollen, painful, and locally hot and red. The pain moved around and became worse on pressure. Yesterday the right knee also became red, painful, and swollen. He developed redness and nodularity in the region of both knees. The rash is not itchy and waxes and wanes.

At present both knee joints are swollen and movement is limited by pain, the right knee being worse than the left. His temperature is 38.2°C and he has a very mild aversion to cold. The patient also complains of headache, sore throat, anorexia, sweating, thirst with a desire to drink, scanty yellow urine, and dry stools. He has been constipated for three days.

The ESR is 80mm/hour. The ECG shows a tachycardia but is otherwise normal.

Tongue

Red body with a slightly yellow coating

Pulse

Rapid and slightly floating

Analysis of symptoms

1. Fever, aversion to cold, and sore throat—invasion by pathogenic factors.
2. Red swollen joints which are hot and painful—obstruction of the channels.
3. Skin rash—pathogenic heat disturbing the blood.
4. Joint pain that migrates and a rash that waxes and wanes—invasion by pathogenic wind.
5. Thirst, sweating, yellow urine, and dry stools—heat consuming the body fluids.
6. Red tongue with yellow coating, rapid pulse—heat.

Basic theory of case

Painful obstruction in the narrow sense implies invasion of the joints by external pathogenic factors. It is characterized by local obstruction of qi and blood leading to joint pain and limitation of movement. The symptoms vary according to the pathogenic factors involved:

1. Wind is the main pathogenic factor which causes wandering (migrating) painful obstruction (also known as wind-predominant painful obstruction).

Wind is often the dominant factor in causing disease, and easily attacks the body. When wind remains in the joints to block the qi and blood circulation, the joints become painful and swollen. Wind is a yang pathogenic factor that characteristically changes and moves. Similarly, the pain and other associated symptoms often change or migrate from place to place.

2. Cold is the main pathogenic factor which causes severe painful obstruction (also known as cold-predominant painful obstruction).

Cold is a yin pathogenic factor that is characterized by constriction and stagnation. When cold attacks the joints the channels and collaterals become constricted and 'freeze' the qi and blood circulation. This causes pain in the joints, and because the cold constricts the channels, the pain does not change but remains fixed and tends to be severe, reflecting the marked constriction.

3. Dampness is the main factor causing fixed painful obstruction (also known as damp-predominant painful obstruction).

Pathogenic dampness is yin and substantial in nature, blocking the circulation of yang qi. When dampness affects the joints the circulation of blood and yang qi is impaired, causing pain in the joints. Dampness is characterized by heaviness and turbidity; the patient may thus complain of heaviness in the joints. The problem is often prolonged.

4. Heat is the main pathogenic factor causing febrile painful obstruction (also known as heat-predominant painful obstruction).

The heat may be external, which directly invades the joint, or it may be from invasion of external wind, cold, or dampness which has transformed into heat. Heat is a yang pathogenic factor which stimulates the circulation of blood, leading to red, swollen, and painful joints. There may be only a local sensation of heat or a systemic fever.

Fig. 3

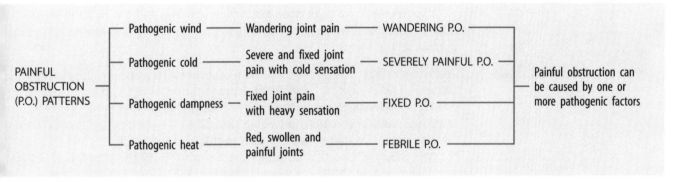

Cause of disease | Wind-heat

In addition to his fever, aversion to cold, headache, and sore throat, the patient also suffers from painful, red, swollen knee and ankle joints. These symptoms indicate invasion by wind-heat. Wind and heat are yang pathogenic factors and thus the symptoms are mainly confined to the surface and upper parts of the body. The joint symptoms are changeable, as is the skin rash, which reflects the moving, changing characteristics of wind, in this case accompanied by obvious signs of heat.

Site of disease | Superficial aspects of the body and the joints

The patient has fever, aversion to cold, a sore throat, and a floating pulse, the principal evidence of involvement of the superficial tissues.

The knee and ankles are red, swollen, and painful with limited movement, thus the joints are involved in the disease.

Pathological change

According to basic theory of painful obstruction, different pathogenic factors may invade the joints and cause different symptoms depending on the factor involved. In the clinical situation, a single factor may cause painful obstruction, but more commonly there is a combination of external pathogenic factors. The diagnosis depends on identifying the key signs and symptoms in order to determine the main cause.

This patient has a clear history of a bad cold with persistent symptoms of fever, aversion to cold, headache, and a sore throat, indicating that the pathogenic factors have attacked the superficial level of the body where they have obstructed the protective qi. The surface of the body has lost the natural warmth of the protective qi, and the patient has accordingly developed an intolerance to cold. The fever, however, is more severe than this mild aversion to cold, as wind-heat is the dominant factor. The patient has a headache and a sore throat, indicating that the yang pathogenic factors have attacked the head and throat where they have caused obstruction.

Soon after the invasion of pathogenic factors the patient began to complain of pain and swelling in the left knee and ankle, followed quickly by involvement of the right knee. This indicates that the wind-heat has blocked the local circulation of qi and blood and affected the joints. The wind causes the pain to move around, while the heat causes the joints to become hot and red. Heat becomes stronger with the passage of time; as the heat symptoms become more severe, the body fluids are consumed. This explains the thirst, sweating, scanty yellow urine, and dry stools.

The patient also has a rash with a circular form which tends to come and go. This is known as erythema annulare or maculopapular rash, *bān zhěn* in traditional Chinese medicine. Wind-heat has disturbed the blood, but not at a very deep level. The transient nature of the rash indicates that wind is the dominant pathogenic factor.

The tongue is red with a slightly yellow coating, and the pulse is rapid and slightly floating. This pulse signifies that the pathogenic factors are still on the surface of the body.

Pattern of disease

In this case there is a combination of an exterior pattern and a channel-collateral pattern. The patient has the general presentation of exterior wind-heat with headache, aversion to cold, fever, sore throat, and a floating pulse. There is also a channel-collateral pattern involving the joints.

The pattern is one of heat, both systemic and localized.

It is excessive because the wind-heat has obstructed the channels and there is no weakness of the antipathogenic factor.

Additional notes

1. Is the heat in this case entirely due to invasion of heat, or is there also some heat from constraint that arose later?

This patient has a clear history of aversion to cold and fever, sore throat, and a floating, rapid pulse. Therefore initially the invasion of wind-heat was the sole cause of the heat pattern. At a later stage, however, the heat symptoms became more severe, indicating the development of heat from constraint. Thus there is evidence to suggest that both causes are involved.

2. Is there any interior pattern involved?

In addition to the exterior pattern this patient does show symptoms of internal heat such as thirst, sweating, scanty yellow urine, dry stools, and a red tongue.

But the heat that is present evolved from the exterior pattern; no particular Organ has yet been involved. In cases such as this, as the external heat is expelled the internal heat will clear.

Conclusion

1. According to the eight principles:
   Exterior and channel-collateral pattern, heat, and excessive pattern.

2. According to etiology:
   Wind-heat invasion.

3. According to channels and collaterals:
   Obstruction of the channels by wind-heat.

Treatment principle

Expel the pathogenic wind and heat.
Cool the blood.
Remove the obstruction from the channels and collaterals and (thereby) alleviate the pain.

Selection of points

G-20 *(feng chi)*   xi yan (M-LE-16)
G-31 *(feng shi)*   he ding (M-LE-27)
Sp-10 *(xue hai)*   B-60 *(kun lun)*
L-11 *(shao shang)*

Explanation of points

G-20 *(feng chi)* has the function of removing pathogenic wind and relieving exterior disorders. It is also used in treating various head symptoms. It can be used to eliminate either wind-cold or wind-heat, and has both local and systemic effects.

G-31 *(feng shi)* removes pathogenic wind and dampness, and relieves obstruction in the channels and collaterals by regulating the qi and blood. It also promotes the proper functioning of the sinews and the channels, especially in the lower limbs. *Feng shi* means 'wind palace', thus this point is effective in removing wind in such disorders as painful obstruction, numbness, paresthesia, and itching. In this case it is chosen specifically to remove the wind-heat.

Sp-10 *(xue hai)* regulates and cools the blood and removes pathogenic wind. This point removes heat from the blood in the entire body, and locally regulates the qi and blood and arrests wind. In this case it also has an important local effect in reducing the swelling and alleviating the pain in the knees.

L-11 *(shao shang)* is the well point of the Lung channel and has a strong effect in clearing heat from the Lung and soothing the throat. The bleeding method is used with a three-edged needle.

xi yan (M-LE-16) are a pair of points below the patella which are indicated for obstruction of the knee joint. They are commonly used in treating problems involving arthritis of the knee, mainly for their local effect. In this case, because the problem is still superficial, the points should not be punctured too deeply, perhaps less than 0.5 inch.

he ding (M-LE-27) is also chosen for its local effect in alleviating pain in the knee and removing obstruction from the joint.

B-60 *(kun lun)* is used to regulate the qi and blood of the ankle joint, reduce swelling, and alleviate pain. It is also a distal point on the foot greater yang channel and can promote the function of the greater yang channel and clear wind-heat from the head and upper parts of the body.

Combination of points

G-20 *(feng chi)* and G-31 *(feng shi)* both belong to the Gallbladder channel and are used to expel wind. One is above and the other is below; together they make a good pair for arresting wind.

xi yan (M-LE-16), Sp-10 *(xue hai)*, and *he ding* (M-LE-27) are an essential group of points for problems of the knee joint. They surround the knee and are effective in removing local obstruction from both the qi and blood in this area.

Follow-up

This patient was treated twice on consecutive days after which his temperature was normal, the aversion to cold had disappeared, and his sore throat was improved. The joints were less swollen and painful, but still painful to touch. He was then treated on alternate days, with L-11 *(shao shang)* no longer being used. After four days the joints continued to improve and he only had pain on flexing the knees more than 90°. Most of the redness and swelling had disappeared, and there was only slight tenderness. His appetite also improved. After two further treatments which included S-36 *(zu san li)*, all the symptoms disappeared and he was able to return to work. At his final treatment only associated points were used to tonify his general energy: B-13 *(fei shu)*, B-20 *(pi shu)*, and B-23 *(shen shu)*. The ESR and ECG were checked twice during treatment, and were within normal limits. He returned for follow-up at six months and one year post-treatment with no recurrence of symptoms.

CASE 25: **Male, age 46**

Main complaint

Pain in right shoulder

History

Three-year history of pain in the right shoulder which has gradually become worse. He was diagnosed as suffering from periarthritis of the shoulder joint. The symptoms worsen with exposure to cold, especially in winter and when the weather is cloudy and damp. Physical labor also exacerbates the pain, and the patient always has difficulty in dressing and undressing. He has tried various remedies including physiotherapy, Western drugs, and Chinese herbs, but with very little success. Because the weather recently turned cold and the pain more severe, he decided to try acupuncture treatment. The patient has no previous health problems and indeed his general health remains good.

On examination there was general tenderness of the deltoid muscle, especially the anterior and upper lateral aspects. There was reduction in the shoulder's range of motion, especially in abduction and internal rotation. There was some atrophy of the muscles of the shoulder girdle on the right.

Tongue

Normal body with a thin white coating

Pulse

Wiry and tight

Analysis of symptoms

1. Tenderness and limited range of motion—obstruction of the channels.
2. Exacerbation of symptoms with changes in the weather—
   invasion of the channels by external pathogenic factors.
3. Wiry, tight pulse—pain.

Basic theory of case

Periarthritis of the shoulder is common in clinical practice, especially in patients of middle age or older. This is also known as fixed or 'frozen' shoulder. As it is common in patients around the age of fifty, it is also called 'fifty shoulder.' The onset is gradual and usually becomes chronic, with the symptoms slowly getting worse. Typical symptoms include pain and limitation of movement of the shoulder with muscular atrophy in the later stages.

After middle age the antipathogenic factor tends to become insufficient and the harmony between nutritive qi and protective qi is lost. It is then more likely that pathogenic factors such as cold, wind, and dampness will invade local areas to cause obstruction of the channels and stagnation of the qi and blood. The onset is so gradual that the patient can rarely recall the initial incident that gave rise to the symptoms. Diagnosis is made on the basis of the symptoms, such as a localized feeling of cold and pain associated with weather change and a preference for heat applied to the shoulder. This disease is painful obstruction in the narrow sense of the term.

Cause of disease

Pathogenic cold

This patient has a three-year history of localized pain in the shoulder related to weather change. The pulse is wiry and tight, indicating a cold pattern.

Site of disease

Shoulder joint

The patient has a fixed pain in the area of the right shoulder.

Pathological change

The patient is approaching fifty years of age, suggesting that when the pathogenic cold invaded the shoulder the local antipathogenic qi was insufficient. The cold therefore remained in the channels and collaterals and caused shoulder pain. Pathogenic cold is characterized by constriction and stagnation and does not move; the pain thus remains localized. The obstruction of the channels is severe because of the constriction, and its associated pain is accordingly severe. Because the original cause of the disease is invasion by external pathogenic factors, when the weather turns cold the pathogenic factor in the channels tends to increase and the symptoms worsen.

Physical labor consumes the body energy and puts more strain on the circulation of qi and blood, which in turn reduces the local flow of qi and blood. Physical stress therefore also makes the pain worse.

The patient has no other symptoms and his general health is good, thus the pathogenic factor has remained in the joint and has not involved any of the Organs. The normal tongue also indicates that the site of disease is not very deep. The pulse is wiry and tight, implying constriction of the vessels by pathogenic cold giving rise to pain.

This patient has a local insufficiency of antipathogenic factor, but does he have a deficiency pattern? In traditional Chinese medicine the onset of any disease must involve a relative deficiency of antipathogenic factor. However, a deficiency pattern is diagnosed on the basis of the entire presentation. In other words, although the onset of disease always involves deficiency of the antipathogenic factor, a pattern of deficiency is not always present. This patient has no symptoms of deficiency in the Organs, just a long history of local pain, which implies that the local channel qi is not strong enough to overcome the invasion of pathogenic cold.

Fig. 4

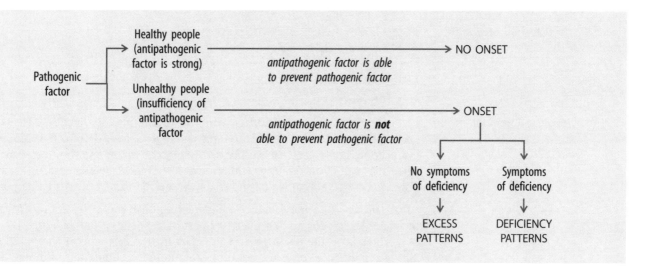

Pattern of disease

There is obstruction of the joint by external pathogenic factors causing obstruction in the channel; it is thus a channel-collateral pattern.

There is no local redness or swelling, and there are no generalized symptoms of heat. Because external cold is the pathogenic factor, this is accordingly a pattern of cold.

The cold is intense and the obstruction in the channel is severe, indicating that the pattern is excessive.

Additional notes

1. Why is cold the only pathogenic factor involved in this case?

Painful obstruction in the narrow sense can be caused by wind, cold, dampness, or heat. In this case there is obviously no heat involved. The pain is fixed so we can exclude the possibility of wind. Cold and dampness both cause fixed pain, but the nature of the pain differs. Cold usually causes severe, aching pain. Dampness mainly causes a feeling of heaviness and stiffness, by comparison to which the pain tends to be mild and sometimes of little significance. This is therefore a typical case of simple cold invasion.

2. Is there any Spleen deficiency in this case?

The Spleen controls the muscles and when there is a Spleen deficiency, especially of Spleen qi, the patient may have muscle wasting. In this case there is localized atrophy of the muscles of the right shoulder girdle, which is quite mild. However, the diagnosis of Spleen deficiency cannot be made according to this symptom as the atrophy in this case is due to limitation of movement by pain and consequent disease. If the circulation of qi and blood in the channel is improved and the pathogenic factor is expelled, the shoulder will be used and the atrophy will improve. If the area involved in atrophy broadens to include the limb, back, or chest wall, and also becomes more severe, a deficiency of Spleen qi would then have to be considered.

Conclusion

1. According to the eight principles:
   Channel-collateral pattern, cold, and excessive.

2. According to etiology:
   Invasion by pathogenic cold.

3. According to channels and collaterals:
   Obstruction of the channels by pathogenic cold, primarily the hand yang brightness Large Intestine channel.

Treatment principle

1. Expel the pathogenic cold and warm the channel.
2. Remove the obstruction from the channel and alleviate the pain.

Selection of points

LI-15 *(jian yu)* right side with warm needle
LI-14 *(bi nao)* right side
jian qian ling (M-UE-48) right side with warm needle
LI-10 *(shou san li)* right side
S-36 *(zu san li)*

Explanation of points

LI-15 *(jian yu)* is a very important point for promoting the function of the shoulder joint and removing obstruction and pathogenic factors from the channels. It is most commonly used for painful obstruction involving the shoulder, especially when the pain is on the upper anterior aspect. When there is cold invasion, the warm needle technique using moxa on the needle can be used at this point.

LI-14 *(bi nao)* is a good choice for removing obstruction from the sinews and the channel. It is located on the lower part of the deltoid. Paired with LI-15 *(jian yu)*, which is on the upper part of this muscle, it makes a good combination for alleviating the local pain and also for promoting the circulation of qi and blood *jian nei ling* (M-UE-48) is located at the mid-point between LI-15 *(jian yu)* and the anterior axillary fold. This miscellaneous point promotes the circulation of qi and blood in the local muscle and shoulder joint. It is an appropriate selection when the symptoms are mainly on the anterior aspect of the shoulder, and especially for limitation of movement.

LI-10 *(shou san li)* is a secondary point for promoting the circulation of qi and blood in the yang brightness channel. Compared to the previous points it is relatively remote and is commonly used in the clinic to promote the circulation of qi and blood and alleviate pain when there is localized obstruction elsewhere along the channel.

S-36 *(zu san li)* is an effective point for promoting the antipathogenic factor and removing obstruction from the channels and collaterals. It is chosen from the foot yang brightness channel to support the hand yang brightness. In this case, both sides would be needled.

Combination of points

LI-15 *(jian yu)*, LI-14 *(bi nao)*, and *jian nei ling* (M-UE-48) are a group of local points used for painful obstruction involving the shoulder. They all promote the function of the joint and sinews, especially on the anterior aspect of the shoulder.

Follow-up

The patient was treated daily, and after one week the pain was obviously reduced in severity. Movement was still very limited, however, especially in trying to raise the arm. There was a local feeling of tightness and any large movement exacerbated the pain. After the first week LI-16 *(ju gu)* was therefore added to the prescription and he was treated on alternate days. After a further two weeks of treatment the feeling of weakness and tension had almost disappeared and the patient could raise his arm a little better. He was then treated twice a week for two more weeks. After five weeks of treatment he was advised to begin gentle and slow exercise of the shoulder, and after six weeks the symptoms had virtually disappeared. He continued exercising and had no recurrence of the shoulder pain.

CASE 26: **Female, age 41**

Main complaint

Joint pain and palpitations

History

The patient has a ten-year history of recurrent episodes of pain in the joints of the upper and lower limbs, especially the small joints of the hand and wrist. The pain in her hands is sometimes so severe that she is unable to move the joints. More recently she has also had pain in the spine. Even though Chinese herbs or acupuncture have controlled the symptoms during each exacerbation, her problem has gradually worsened.

During the last year she has had low energy and developed palpitations and dyspnea on exertion. She has no chest pain but does have a stifling sensation in the chest. Her symptoms improve with rest. At times when all the symptoms are severe, she has edema of the lower limbs with some pitting at the ankles. The edema is absent in the mornings and becomes more obvious during the day. She sleeps poorly and does not like to drink, but her appetite is normal. Her urine is reduced in quantity, but her bowels are normal.

Tongue

Normal body color with a thin, white, moist coating

Pulse

Soft and rather rapid

Analysis of symptoms

1. Recurrent joint pain—obstruction of the channels.
2. Reduced energy, palpitations and dyspnea on exertion—Heart qi deficiency.

3. Stifling sensation in the chest—qi obstruction in the upper burner.

4. Edema of the lower limbs with no desire to drink and reduced urine output—retention of harmful water.

5. Moist, white tongue coating—damp-cold.

6. Soft pulse—dampness.

Basic theory of case

Painful obstruction in the general sense includes that of the yin Organs, with symptoms based upon which of the yin Organs is affected.

1. Lung painful obstruction: wheezing and a stifling sensation in the chest, or shortness of breath. Symptoms are always worse on exertion.

2. Heart painful obstruction: palpitations, anxiety, and a heavy, stifling sensation in the chest. The palpitations may be very severe and the patient may be restless and upset, in part because the patient is aware of the pounding of her heart.

3. Spleen painful obstruction: weakness of the limbs, hiccup, vomiting, nausea, and anorexia.

4. Liver painful obstruction: stifling sensation in the costal and hypochondriac regions. Some patients feel a mass in the epigastrium. Poor sleep with a tendency to wake up with a start.

5. Kidney painful obstruction: muscular weakness or atrophy of the limbs and weakness of the spinal column with difficulty in standing for long periods or walking. Some patients feel so weak that they are reluctant to get up.

On the basis of symptoms alone, the patterns of painful obstruction in the five yin Organs are difficult to distinguish from other disorders of the yin Organs. For example, invasion of the Lung by pathogenic factors or Lung qi deficiency can give rise to symptoms similar to those described as Lung painful obstruction. Liver qi stagnation or Liver yin or blood deficiency may likewise resemble Liver painful obstruction. The key to diagnosis lies in a history of previous joint pain, usually of rather long duration. Painful obstruction of the five yin Organs starts with an invasion of the joints by some combination of the external pathogenic factors wind, cold, and dampness. After a period of time, these pathogenic factors pass from the joints through the channels into one or more of the yin Organs. Painful obstruction of the yin Organs therefore fits into the category of invasion by external pathogenic factors, but is not an exterior pattern.

Fig. 5

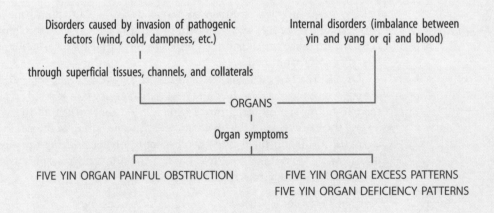

Disorders caused by invasion of pathogenic factors (wind, cold, dampness, etc.)   Internal disorders (imbalance between yin and yang or qi and blood)

through superficial tissues, channels, and collaterals

ORGANS

Organ symptoms

FIVE YIN ORGAN PAINFUL OBSTRUCTION   FIVE YIN ORGAN EXCESS PATTERNS
FIVE YIN ORGAN DEFICIENCY PATTERNS

Cause of disease

Pathogenic cold

The main complaint is one of pain in the joints of the limbs and spinal column. The pain does not wander, and there are no symptoms of heaviness or a feverish sensation. This indicates that cold has invaded and caused obstruction of the channels. The pain here is typical of invasion by cold.

Site of disease

The joints and Heart

There is an obvious problem in the joints of the limbs and spine.

The palpitations, dyspnea, poor sleep, and stifling sensation in the chest indicate that the Heart is involved.

Pathological change

The main pathological change in this case is blockage of the joints by pathogenic factors, which after a long period of time have affected the yin Organ. Cold has obstructed the channels, leading to poor circulation of qi and blood in the joints and consequently joint pain. After each episode of pain, although the symptoms disappear with treatment, some cold remains in the joints, thus the disease is recurrent and the symptoms gradually worsen.

During the past year the patient has had palpitations and a stifling sensation in the chest with poor sleep. This indicates that the cold has passed from the joints into the channels, and then to the Heart. Cold is a yin pathogenic factor which can injure the yang qi of the body. In this case the Heart qi has been weakened, thus the patient complains of palpitations and dyspnea. The spirit has been deprived of its normal nourishment, thus the patient's sleep is disturbed.

Because the Heart qi is deficient, the pectoral qi *(zōng qì)* has become stagnant, leading to a stifling sensation in the chest. The edema is caused by a disorder of water metabolism and always appears when the symptoms affecting the chest are at their worst. The stagnation of pectoral qi has given rise to edema through its effects on the water pathways. There is retention of harmful water and dampness, which accounts for the lack of thirst, edema, and reduced output of urine.

The tongue body is normal in color, meaning that the disease is still at the qi level and has not influenced the blood. The white, moist tongue coating and soft pulse signify retention of cold and dampness.

Pattern of disease

This patient has a combination of a channel-collateral and an interior pattern. The cold has obstructed the joints, which causes pain, and has also affected the Heart qi, which causes the other symptoms.

This pattern is one of pure cold. There are no symptoms of heat.

It is also a combination of excess and deficiency. Excess is reflected in the joint pain caused by obstruction of the channels by pathogenic cold, and also in the retention of harmful water which has resulted in edema. Deficiency is reflected in the chest, where there is shortness of breath.

Additional notes

1. Why is the pulse rather rapid, and is this a sign of heat?

A rapid pulse usually indicates the presence of heat, but in this case the pulse is also forceless. The Heart qi deficiency leads to a reduction in the force of the Heart beat, thus the rate increases to produce a normal cardiac output. There is accordingly no heat mechanism involved.

2. Is there a Lung disorder in this case?

The Lungs, situated in the upper burner, are also responsible for water metabolism. The Heart qi deficiency has affected the pectoral qi, which inevitably has also affected the Lungs to some extent, but there are no symptoms relating to the Lungs. Edema in this case occurs only when the Heart symptoms are severe, so there is no basis on which to diagnose a Lung problem.

3. What is the crucial difference between this case and case number 23?

In both cases there is a history of joint pain with Heart symptoms, including palpitations, stifling sensation in the chest, and poor sleep. In this case, however, there is also a clear history of chronic joint pain followed eventually by Heart painful obstruction. In case number 23 this relationship is not present.

Conclusion

1. According to the eight principles:
   Combination of channel-collateral and interior pattern, cold, and a combination of excess and deficiency.
2. According to etiology:
   Invasion by pathogenic cold.
3. According to channels and collaterals:
   Obstruction and constriction of the channels by pathogenic cold (severe painful obstruction).
4. According to Organ theory:
   Heart qi injury (Heart painful obstruction).

Treatment principle

1. Expel the pathogenic cold and remove the obstruction from the channels to alleviate pain.
2. Tonify the Heart qi and calm the spirit.

Selection of points

P-4 *(xi men)*   B-13 *(fei shu)*
LI-4 *(he gu)*   B-15 *(xin shu)*
GV-14 *(da zhui)*   S-36 *(zu san li)*
GV-9 *(zhi yang)*

Explanation of points

P-4 *(xi men)* is effective in calming the spirit. It is the accumulating point of the Pericardium channel and can remove obstruction from the chest, especially when there is severe chest pain, palpitations, and a stifling sensation. Locally it also treats elbow and wrist pain, as it is situated near the mid-point of the forearm, and effectively removes obstruction from the channel.

LI-4 *(he gu)* is good for expelling pathogenic wind and relieving exterior patterns. It removes obstruction from the channels and eases pain, especially in the hands. Use a needle at least 2 units in length, threading in the direction of P-8 *(lao gong)*. Warm needle technique with moxa is used to expel the pathogenic cold.

GV-14 *(da zhui)* is a meeting point of all the yang channels and is used mainly to remove obstruction from the governing vessel, since the patient has pain in the spine. It therefore functions to remove obstruction, treat local pain, and also strengthen the antipathogenic factor by drawing on the energy from all the yang channels. The method of manipulation should accordingly be balanced to achieve the dual goals of dispersing and tonifying.

GV-9 *(zhi yang)* on the governing vessel removes the stifling sensation from the chest and regulates the qi. It is below T7 and has a strong local effect in alleviating pain in the spine and strengthening the Heart qi.

B-13 *(fei shu)* tonifies the Lung qi and promotes the Lung functions of descending and dispersing, hence arresting asthma.

B-15 *(xin shu)* treats symptoms involving the Heart, calms the spirit, and harmonizes the nutritive and the protective qi.

B-13 *(fei shu)* and B-15 *(xin shu)* are both used because the problem is mainly in the upper burner; they remove the painful obstruction of the Heart caused by cold, and also help regulate water metabolism in the upper burner, thus reducing the edema.

S-36 *(zu san li)* strengthens the antipathogenic factor and removes obstruction from the channels in the lower limbs to alleviate pain.

Follow-up

The patient was treated on alternate days. After four treatments the stifling sensation in the chest and shortness of breath were much improved. The palpitations occurred only occasionally. The pain in the spine was almost completely relieved, and there was no edema. The patient was sleeping well. The pain in the small joints of the hands was slightly less severe. The patient received three further treatments, after which she was symptom-free.

In view of her chronic history, she was advised to use a moxa stick above the joints and also at S-36 *(zu san li)* every day for three months. She was also prescribed the Chinese herbal formula, Emperor of Heaven's Special Pill to Tonify the Heart *(tian wang bu xin dan)*, to help restore her general energy. At the end of this time she had no palpitations or edema and her general energy was good. She had only fleeting pain in the joints, which did not interfere with her daily life, and she was happy to continue with moxa at home for an additional three months. After this time her condition remained satisfactory.

CASE 27: **Male, age 14**

Main complaint

Pain on the left lower neck and shoulder

History

This child had two cycling accidents in recent years. Three months ago he was taking part in a race and again fell off his bicycle onto his left side while cycling at high speed. He felt pain on the left side of his neck and the posterior and upper aspects of the left shoulder. The pain was worse on moving the shoulder joint, and the symptoms were still present after three months. When he tries to cycle he has aching from the shoulder to the wrist with some numbness of the anterior aspect of the forearm.

At the time of the accident he was X-rayed and there was no bone injury or displacement. The diagnosis was whiplash injury to the cervical spine with soft tissue injury to the shoulder. He was treated with physiotherapy and local cortisone injections. He also saw a chiropractor and took homeopathic remedies, but the symptoms persisted. His general health is good.

On examination there was slight swelling on the left side of the neck with tenderness on the left side of the spinous process of C7. The posterior and superior aspects of the left shoulder were tender. He was unable to raise his left arm anteriorly more than 140°. His right shoulder movements were normal.

Tongue

Normal body, thin white coating

Pulse

Slightly wiry

Analysis of symptoms

1. History of recurrent injury—blood stasis from trauma.
2. Pain on the nape and shoulder with limitation of movement— obstruction in the channels.
3. Numbness —malnourishment of the channel.
4. Wiry pulse—pain.

Basic theory of case

Painful obstruction of blood is usually considered to be obstruction or blood stasis in the channels as a result of exposure to wind, and possibly also cold and dampness.[1] This may occur during sleep or after heavy physical exertion, which causes profuse sweating. The main symptoms are pain in the limbs and joints, numbness or paresthesia of the limbs, and a choppy pulse. The basic pathological change

---

1. The other condition referred to by this name is characterized by localized numbness, parasthesia, and pain that moves. This condition is due to either externally-contracted wind or excessive sweating upon exercise in patients with qi and blood deficiency. This definition of blood painful obstruction goes back to the *Essentials from the Golden Cabinet*.

is poor circulation of blood leading to malnourishment of the muscles and skin. The essential problem is blood stasis; accordingly, in the clinical situation joint pain caused by blood stasis is generally referred to as blood painful obstruction. This category includes both trauma and the invasion of pathogenic factors which cause blood stasis. Some patients who exhibit these symptoms have no history of precipitating factors; they are also included in this group.

Cause of disease

Blood stasis

There is a clear history of trauma and the symptoms are local pain, swelling and numbness of the arm, all indicating injury of the local vessels resulting in impairment of blood circulation.

Site of disease

Joints

The injury is mainly on the left nape and shoulder, with limitation of movement of the left shoulder. The joints of the cervical spine and shoulder are therefore involved.

Pathological change

Because this patient has no history of exposure to pathogenic factors, this is an obvious example of blood painful obstruction caused by trauma. The injury involved the nape of the neck and shoulder, with local blood stasis causing swelling. The channels are obstructed and the circulation of qi and blood is impaired, causing severe pain and limitation of movement.

When blood stagnates, its normal function of nourishing the tissues is impaired, as is its local circulation; this can lead to numbness. The site of disease is localized and has not influenced the Organs, thus there are no general symptoms of disease.

The tongue is normal, indicating that the general qi and blood, and yin and yang, has not been affected. The wiry pulse is an indication of pain.

Fig. 6

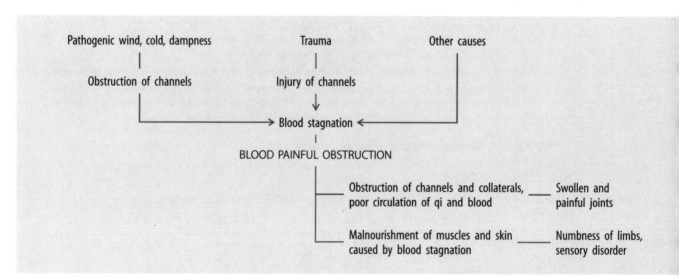

Pathogenic wind, cold, dampness   Trauma   Other causes

Obstruction of channels   Injury of channels

Blood stagnation

BLOOD PAINFUL OBSTRUCTION

Obstruction of channels and collaterals, poor circulation of qi and blood —— Swollen and painful joints

Malnourishment of muscles and skin caused by blood stagnation —— Numbness of limbs, sensory disorder

Pattern of disease

This is a channel-collateral pattern since the symptoms are confined to the channels.

There is neither heat nor cold.

There is blood stasis and the antipathogenic factor is unaffected; it is thus a pattern of excess.

Additional notes

What is the relationship between painful obstruction caused by wind, cold, or dampness and blood painful obstruction?

When pathogenic factors invade the joint and thereby obstruct the channel, this may lead to a common type of painful obstruction (wandering painful obstruction, severe painful obstruction, and fixed painful obstruction). However, if the obstruction becomes intense, there will then be blood stasis and a pattern of blood painful obstruction will ensue. In the clinical situation, the pain will be more severe, numbness is usually noted, and the pulse may become choppy.

When there is a history of trauma a diagnosis of blood painful obstruction can be made at the time of the initial injury if no other factors are present. Some patients present with a history of previous trauma followed by invasion of pathogenic factors, and in such cases the diagnosis will depend on the entire presentation.

Conclusion

1. According to the eight principles:
   Channel-collateral pattern; neither cold nor heat; excessive pattern.

2. According to etiology:
   Blood stasis.

3. According to channels and collaterals:
   Blood stasis in the channels (blood painful obstruction).

Treatment principle

1. Remove the obstruction in the channels and disperse the swelling.
2. Alleviate pain.

Selection of points

hua tuo jia ji (M-BW-35) at C7 (left side only)
LI-15 *(jian yu)*
SI-11 *(tian zong)*
G-21 *(jian jing)*
LI-12 *(zhou liao)*
S-38 *(tiao kou)* through to B-57 *(cheng shan)*

Explanation of points

Hua tuo jia ji (M-BW-35): There were originally seventeen pairs of *jia ji* (M-BW-35) points from T1 to L5. They are called Hua Tuo's *jia ji* (M-BW-35) points because their discovery is attributed to that famous later Han physician. These points brought good therapeutic results and were safe to use in the clinic; their number has therefore been extended to points in the neck from C4 to C7, the method of location being the same. They are very useful in treating whiplash injuries, cervical spondylosis, and other painful problems of the neck. They can be used individually, as a pair, or as a group. The one by C7 was used in this case as a local point to remove obstruction, promote the circulation of qi and blood, and alleviate pain.

LI-15 *(jian yu)* promotes the function of the shoulder joint, alleviates pain, and is especially useful for treating symptoms on the superior and anterior aspects of the shoulder, including the inability to raise the arm fully, as in this case.

SI-11 *(tian zong)* is effective in removing pathogenic factors and obstruction from the channels. It is located on the scapula and is a good local point for relieving symptoms occurring on the posterior aspect of the shoulder. It also removes obstruction on the hand greater yang channel, and will therefore relieve pain and numbness in the arm and forearm.

G-21 *(jian jing)* regulates the qi and removes obstruction from the lesser yang channels. Here it will help with the limitation of movement caused by pain on the posterior aspect of the shoulder.

LI-12 *(zhou liao)* regulates the qi and promotes the function of the joint by relaxing the sinews. When combined with LI-15 *(jian yu)* it regulates the entire hand yang brightness channel to alleviate pain and remove numbness below the shoulder.

S-38 *(tiao kou)* through to B-57 *(cheng shan)*: S-38 *(tiao kou)* relaxes the sinews and regulates the qi, and in this case the foot yang brightness channel qi is directed to the foot greater yang, as the symptoms and hence the obstruction are more severe in the greater yang channel. This method uses the foot channels to treat a hand channel disorder. The point is used in this way as a result of long clinical experience.

Combination of points

SI-11 *(tian zong)* and G-21 *(jian jing)*, one point on the Small Intestine channel and the other on the Gallbladder channel, are located on the back of the shoulder, one above and one below. The channels pass in a horizontal direction along the top of the shoulder to the nape of the neck, and vertically between these two points. The combination of these points accordingly influences a large local area. SI-11 *(tian zong)* primarily removes stagnation and obstruction, while G-21 *(jian jing)* especially regulates the qi.

Follow-up

After one treatment the patient said that the shoulder pain and forearm numbness were improved. The pain in the nape and anterior upper arm remained severe. He was treated twice during the following week, after which the swelling on the nape of the neck disappeared. He then complained of pain on the anterior edge of the deltoid muscle, and the point *jian qian ling* (M-UE-48) was therefore added. He was then treated once a week. After two more weeks all his symptoms had disappeared. He took part in a cycle race soon afterward with no ill-effects; in fact, he won the race and received a gold medal.

CASE 28: **Female, age 46**

Main complaint

Pain in both elbows

History

This patient has a rural background. She is accustomed to hard physical labor and to carrying heavy loads for a considerable distance. Four months ago she carried a heavy weight of books for several hours to reach a bus-stop. The same evening both her elbows became very painful. The symptoms did not improve with rest, and since that time she has been unable to carry anything without severe pain, especially in the right elbow.

The original injury occurred during the winter but she does not associate the symptoms with cold weather. Local heat and massage have no effect on the pain. The patient is obese but has previously enjoyed excellent health. Her appetite, sleep pattern, bowels, and urine are normal.

On examination there is obvious tenderness on the lateral epicondyles of the humerus, worse on the right side, with bilateral local muscle tenderness.

Tongue

Normal color with a thin and slightly yellow coating

Pulse

Sunken and moderate

Analysis of symptoms

1. History of carrying a heavy weight for a long period—injury to the local tissues.

2. Joint pain—obstruction of the channel.

3. Sunken, moderate pulse—poor circulation of qi and blood in the vessels.

Basic theory of case

In Chinese medicine, stress *(láo,* also known as consumption) is considered to be an important cause of disease. There are three types of stress: *ti lao* or physical stress, *nao lao* or mental stress, and *fang lao* or sexual stress, when either the individuals have very different levels of sexual need, or when both indulge in excessive sexual activity over a prolonged period. Generally speaking, these three types of stress are believed to cause internal disorders, but the pathological change and effect on the Organs is different in each case.

Physical stress which occurs over a long period of time means that the antipathogenic factor is eventually depleted, as there is never time for full recovery to occur after its consumption. The antipathogenic factor will become injured and disease will occur. A sudden burst of intense physical activity can also have the same result, especially in a person with a weak constitution. The pathological change in the case of physical stress is consumption of qi, which leads to an imbalance of yin and yang as well as qi and blood, causing various disorders.

Among the Organs it is most commonly the Spleen that is affected, as the Spleen controls the muscles and is responsible for producing qi and blood. In its early stages, physical stress may give rise to symptoms such as lassitude and poor appetite. In its later stages these can become very severe, and the patient may become emaciated. Other Organs may be affected by different kinds of physical stress, e.g., too much talking may injure the Lung qi and result in a reluctance to speak and shortness of breath. People who have to stand for long periods of time may injure the qi of the Kidneys, and may complain of weakness of the lower limbs and aching in the bones.

Cause of disease

Physical stress

The patient has a long history of carrying heavy loads, and the pain now is exacerbated when she attempts to carry anything.

Site of disease

Joints

The patient has pain in both elbows, which is fixed in one place; thus only these joints are involved.

Pathological change

This case belongs to a mild pattern of painful obstruction of the sinews. Sinews and ligaments are mainly located in the vicinity of joints, and joints are known in Chinese medicine as 'the palace of the sinews' *(jīn zhī fǔ)*. The sinews are nourished by qi and blood and facilitate the movement of the muscles.

This patient has a long history of carrying heavy loads, thus the local qi and blood had become weakened and the function in the elbows had gradually diminished. When she carried a particularly heavy load she consumed even more qi and blood. The undernourished sinews became overworked, injuring the elbows and causing constant pain for four months. It is because of this injury to the elbows that the symptoms become worse when she now attempts to carry anything.

There is no invasion by pathogenic factors, only the local injury, so the pain is not related to change in the weather. The local application of heat and massage is too superficial and does not improve the deep injury to the sinews. Her general health is good, thus the yin and yang, qi and blood are still normal.

Pattern of disease

This is a channel-collateral pattern. The physical stress has caused injury to the joints and sinews with no invasion by pathogenic factors.

The system of channels and collaterals includes the regular channels, the eight extra channels, divergent channels and collaterals, the tendinomuscular channel, and the cutaneous regions. Channel-collateral patterns therefore encompass a wide range of disorders.

There is no obvious heat or cold in this particular pattern.

There is some local injury to the qi, but as pain is the main problem, the pattern is one of excess.

Additional notes

1. What is the significance of the tongue and pulse?

This patient has a long history of obesity, implying accumulation of dampness and phlegm. The tongue coating is slightly yellow, as this type of problem has a tendency to transform into heat. The tongue body is normal in color, suggesting that the heat is very mild and has yet to become significant. (There are no other heat-related symptoms.) The sunken, moderate pulse indicates internal accumulation of dampness.

2. Is there a Liver problem in this case?

The Liver controls the sinews, which in this case have been injured. However, there is no Liver blood deficiency, and the problem is very localized and caused only by physical stress. There are no other symptoms associated with the Liver, and thus it is not involved.

3. Is there Spleen qi deficiency?

There are no symptoms relating to the digestive system, but the patient has a long history of physical stress and accumulation of dampness and phlegm. This is confirmed by the tongue and pulse signs. Spleen function is thus somewhat diminished. The problem is not sufficiently severe to be diagnosed as Spleen qi deficiency, but this could be considered in terms of treatment.

Fig. 7

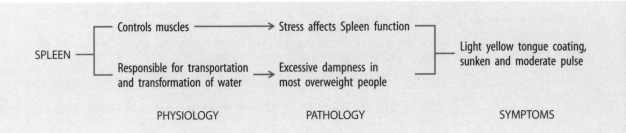

SPLEEN	Controls muscles	→ Stress affects Spleen function	Light yellow tongue coating, sunken and moderate pulse
	Responsible for transportation and transformation of water	→ Excessive dampness in most overweight people	
	PHYSIOLOGY	PATHOLOGY	SYMPTOMS

Conclusion

1. According to the eight principles:
   Channel-collateral pattern; neither heat nor cold; pattern of excess.

2. According to etiology:
   Physical stress causing injury to the sinews.

3. According to channels and collaterals:
   Obstruction of the channel (painful obstruction of the sinews).

Treatment principle

1. Remove the obstruction from the channels.
2. Relax the sinews.
3. Tonify the Spleen.

Selection of points

LI-12 *(zhou liao)*
LI-10 *(shou san li)*
Ashi points
S-36 *(zu san li)*
Sp-9 *(yin ling quan)*

Explanation of points

LI-12 *(zhou liao)* is a point which relaxes the sinews and alleviates pain, its function here being mainly to promote the local circulation of qi and blood and the function of the joint. It will help alleviate pain from the elbow and arm.

LI-10 *(shou san li)* alleviates pain and swelling from the local muscles and promotes the circulation of qi and blood around the channel.

Ashi points are used primarily to remove obstruction from the painful areas.

S-36 *(zu san li)* regulates the function of the Spleen and Stomach and promotes the antipathogenic factor. It is primarily used in this case to treat the chronic weakness of the Spleen.

Sp-9 *(yin ling quan)* tonifies the Spleen and removes dampness.

Combination of points

LI-12 *(zhou liao)* and S-36 *(zu san li)* remove obstruction from the elbow, especially from the yang brightness channel. The warm needle technique can be used on both points to promote the movement of qi around the channel. This pair of points is commonly used in the clinic for elbow pain.

Follow-up

The patient was treated four times during a two-week period. After the first treatment the right elbow was much improved, the left elbow remaining tender at the Ashi points. After two further treatments the elbows had completely recovered, but she had again been working hard and there was tenderness in the muscles on the left side. She received one more treatment after which she was symptom-free. At follow-up two months later there were no apparent symptoms.

Diagnostic principles for painful obstruction

Concept of Painful Obstruction

In Chinese medicine the term *bì* means obstruction of qi and blood. The concept of painful obstruction is therefore extremely broad, and in the clinical situation the symptoms can be quite varied. Painful obstruction patterns can also be classified in various ways, as shown below.

1. According to etiology:

   Wandering painful obstruction (wind-predominant painful obstruction)
   Severe painful obstruction (cold-predominant painful obstruction)
   Fixed painful obstruction (damp-predominant painful obstruction)
   Febrile painful obstruction (heat-predominant painful obstruction)

2. According to depth of disease:

   Skin painful obstruction
   Muscle painful obstruction
   Vessel painful obstruction
   Sinew painful obstruction
   Bone painful obstruction

3. According to disorders of the (yin) Organs:

   Heart painful obstruction
   Lung painful obstruction
   Spleen painful obstruction
   Liver painful obstruction
   Kidney painful obstruction

4. According to the site of the symptoms:

   Chest painful obstruction (with chest pain and a stifling sensation)
   Throat painful obstruction (with hoarseness, pain, and swelling of the pharynx)
   Bladder painful obstruction (with retention of urine)

In addition, there are patterns such as painful obstruction of the qi, blood, and food. Painful obstruction of food, for example, covers all the symptoms associated with dysphagia as well as intestinal obstruction; it is thus not a very useful term, being too broad. In modern Chinese medical practice the term *yē gé* is used for esophageal obstruction, and *fǎn wèi* for obstruction of the Stomach or duodenum. Some types of painful obstruction can be called by two or more names. For example, painful obstruction of the Lung is the same as painful obstruction of qi, and painful obstruction of the vessels is the same as painful obstruction of blood.

Etiology and Pathology of Painful Obstruction Patterns

There are two principal causes of painful obstruction, the most common being invasion by external pathogenic factors, and the less common being internal imbalance. The external factors are wind, cold, dampness, and heat, which can invade the body individually or in combination. There are many causes of internal imbalance which may lead to painful obstruction, among them blood stasis, retention of dampness and phlegm, and injury to qi and blood or the antipathogenic factor.

Irrespective of the precipitating cause, painful obstruction means pathological obstruction of the channels and collaterals or qi stagnation and blood stasis, all of which lead to pain. The channels are connected to the Organs in an interior-exterior relationship. After a period of time, a problem affecting the channels may therefore affect the Organs, qi, and blood and the pattern may thus change to a more complex form of painful obstruction.

Fig. 8

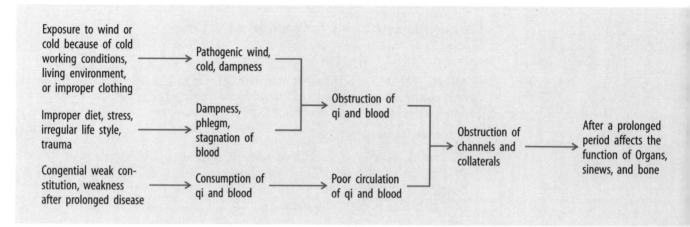

Procedure of Diagnosis in Painful Obstruction

The first step in diagnosis is to determine the cause of obstruction, and to judge the degree of injury to the antipathogenic factor. Most patterns are excessive, i.e., there is invasion by pathogenic factors; patterns of deficiency are generally of less importance.

Secondly, it is necessary to determine the site of the disease, which will be quite evident when the obstruction is in the channels or at the qi or blood level. The site of pain is the site of disease. If the Organs are involved there will be general symptoms, and Organ differentiation should be followed in the usual way. *See Fig. 9, next page.*

Fig. 9

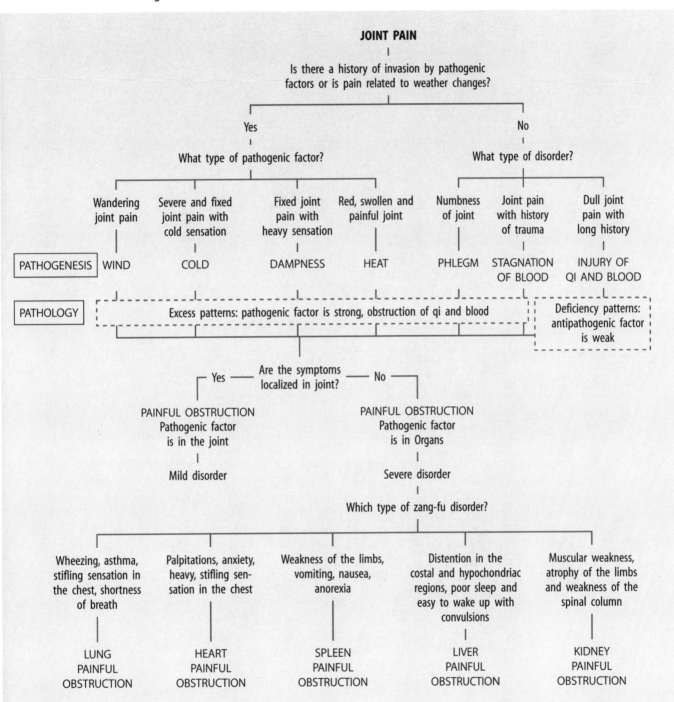

Windstroke

CASE 29: **Female, age 49**

Main complaint

Deviation of mouth and eye

History

One week ago after sleeping in a draft, the patient awoke with this problem which was accompanied by the following symptoms: right-side headache, discomfort at the top of the head, sore, pounding sensation in the right eye, inability to close the right eye and copious watery discharge from the eye.

On examination, when the patient attempts to close her right eye, a small gap of 2mm remains. Wrinkles on the right side of the forehead have disappeared. The right side nasolabial fold has become distinctly less pronounced and the right angle of the mouth has dropped. When the patient was asked to smile in order to reveal her teeth, four were visible on the left but only two on the right. The patient's blood pressure was 90 over 60mmHg. Since onset of the paralysis she has also had episodic palpitations, difficulty in falling asleep, and a bitter taste in the mouth. The patient is not thirsty and has slightly dry stool. Her appetite and urination are normal.

Tongue

The body of the tongue is slightly redder than normal, the coating is very light yellow and is a little bit thicker than usual.

Pulse

The pulse is soft on both sides, but the right side is a bit more sunken.

Analysis of symptoms

1. Right-sided facial paralysis (disappearance of forehead wrinkles, inability to close the right eye, diminishment of the nasolabial fold, and deviation of the mouth)—obstruction of the channels and collaterals.

2. Headache, distention of the right eye—invasion and obstruction of collaterals by pathogenic wind.

3. Palpitations, insomnia, bitter taste in the mouth, and dry stool—heat.

4. Slightly red tongue, light yellow coating—heat.

5. Sunken pulse on right side—obstruction of qi.

Basic theory of case

In traditional Chinese medicine, windstroke is expressed as a group of some or all of the following symptoms: deviation of the eyes and mouth, hemiplegia, a sudden bout of unconsciousness. Its etiology revolves around the presence of internal or external wind. Just as in the environment where wind can gust viciously without warning and then disappear, the onset of this disorder is always sudden and its symptoms often quickly change. Traditional Chinese medicine divides windstroke into four patterns:

1. Collateral pattern

This pattern of windstroke, the mildest of the four types, involves an attack on the collaterals alone. As branches of the channels, the collaterals are most closely associated with the superficial aspects of the body. When wind injures the collaterals, the symptoms are mild and localized, e.g., deviation of the eye and mouth, slight motor impairment, or partial numbness or paresthesia. The patient may or may not have other mild symptoms of discomfort.

2. Channel pattern

This pattern of windstroke involves an attack on the channels. It is more severe than the collateral type because the injury has occurred on a deeper level; its symptoms are thus more widespread, e.g., monoplegia, hemiplegia, and obvious disorder of sensation. Usually the patient will have accompanying symptoms of general ill health, including poor digestion, insomnia, and fatigue.

In both the collateral and channel patterns of windstroke, only the qi and blood circulation has been affected. There has been no injury to the Organs themselves. The spirit remains clear and neither of these types ever occurs with loss of consciousness.

3. Yang Organ pattern

The yang Organ pattern of windstroke is severe. The combination of excessive internal wind with phlegm and blood stasis greatly disturbs the circulation of qi and blood throughout the body. Consequently the principal functions of the spirit and the Organs are often greatly disrupted. Typical manifestations of this pattern are loss of consciousness, hemiplegia, aphasia, and other signs of a serious disorder such as rough breathing with a gurgling sound in the throat, trismus, rigid limbs, red complexion, intense abdominal distention, retention of urine and stool, a deep red tongue with a greasy, yellow coating, and a slippery pulse that is also forceful, rapid, or both.

4. Yin Organ pattern

This is the most severe stage of windstroke. In this pattern the pathogenic factors are extremely strong and the antipathogenic factor is very fragile and precarious. The qi of the yin Organs is near collapse. This means that the antipathogenic factor is beginning to float. If allowed to further develop, the yin and yang of the body will separate, which is one definition of death in traditional Chinese medicine. In addition to some of the main symptoms of yang Organ-type windstroke, e.g., unconsciousness and paralysis, there will also be evidence of collapsing yin or yang. Both types of collapse exhibit very weak and shallow breathing, flaccid muscle tone, and incontinence of urine and stool. With yang collapse there is also cold limbs and body, profuse and cold sweat, a pale tongue with a white coating, and a frail pulse. Collapse of yin is manifested by profuse and warm sweat, a red and dry tongue, and a frail and rapid pulse.

Both the yin and yang Organ patterns have poorer prospects for recovery than the channel and collateral patterns of windstroke. The major distinguishing symptoms of the yin and yang Organ patterns are loss of consciousness and hemiplegia. Because the antipathogenic factor is blocked by the pathogenic factors in the yang Organ type, it is known as the closed type *(bì zhèng);* and because such patients have a very tense musculature, it is also known as the tense or tonic type. In the yin Organ pattern the antipathogenic factor is collapsing and abandoning the body; it is thus known as the abandoned type *(tuō zhèng)*. Because these patients also have a very flaccid musculature, it is also referred to as the flaccid type.

Cause of disease	Pathogenic wind

This particular patient has a clear history of exposure to pathogenic wind. The right-side facial paralysis is proof that the wind has invaded the collaterals in this area, and that the qi and blood circulation there has been disrupted.

Site of disease	Collaterals

The collaterals at the right side of the face have been affected. This is shown by the fact that the wrinkles on the patient's forehead and the nasolabial fold have become more shallow, and the mouth and eye are deviated.

Pathological change

The collateral pattern represents the mildest form of windstroke. The patient may or may not have a history of exposure to external pathogenic factors, but the affected areas will be those which are most vulnerable to exposure, like the face and limbs.

In this case the patient has clearly suffered from exposure to pathogenic wind. The pathogenic factor has disrupted the collaterals on the face, and qi and blood circulation has been obstructed. This is the cause of the patient's migraine and distending sensation of the eye. The channels and collaterals transport qi and blood which nourish the muscles and skin. Because the pathogenic factors have obstructed this system, the muscles and skin have become loose and weak, resulting in shallowness of the wrinkles on the forehead and the nasolabial fold. The weakness of the eye with increased lachrymation has been brought about by the same process.

Wind is a yang pathogenic factor; after it has entered the body it can easily cause heat to develop. This process is facilitated by the presence of stagnant qi and blood in the channels and collaterals. The patient has a one-week history of illness. Initially the pathogenic factor only affected the outer surface of the body, but then a new pattern of heat from stagnation arose. The bitter taste in the mouth and the dry stool clearly indicate that there is heat in the interior. Palpitations and insomnia are symptoms of heat disturbing the spirit. This patient, however, is not thirsty which suggests that the heat is not yet strong enough to consume the fluids.

The tongue is slightly redder than normal, with a thin yellow coating. This would indicate that the heat is mild, but if left untreated it may develop further. In broad terms a sunken pulse indicates a disorder of the Organs, but in this case the pulse is only slightly sunken. This is due to the pathogenic factors residing in the superficial layers of the body where they prevent the yang qi from reaching *Fig. 1* these areas.

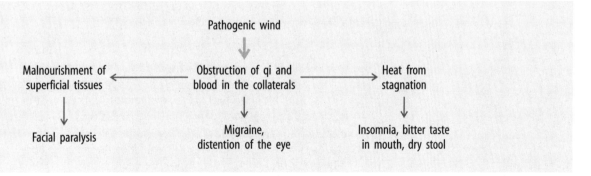

In the basic theory of the case (see above) we explained how to distinguish mild from severe windstroke. The diagnosis is reached by determining whether the spirit and Organs have been affected. While this case is an example of the mildest type (collateral pattern) of windstroke, the patient also exhibits some related problems

Fig. 2

in her general health; however, these are not significant as both the signs and symptoms are quite mild. In patterns of severe windstroke the yin or yang Organs and spirit would be directly attacked by the excessive pathogenic factor or factors, and the symptoms would be more intense.

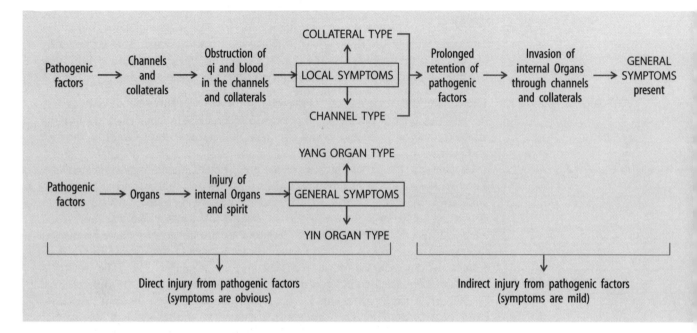

Pattern of disease

In this case the external pathogenic factors have disrupted the local collaterals and progressed to a mild disturbance of the Organs. Hence this patient exhibits a type of channel-collateral pattern, along with a mild interior pattern.

The bitter taste in the mouth, dry stools, palpitations, and red tongue with a yellow coating are clear indications of a heat pattern.

The short history of illness, excessive pathogenic factors, obstruction of the collaterals, and absence of deficiency reveal a pattern of pure excess.

Additional notes

1. Which collaterals have been attacked by the pathogenic wind?

The patient told us that her discomfort was on the side of the head and the face. These two areas are governed by the lesser yang and yang brightness channels respectively. The wind has injured the collaterals of these channels, which allowed the heat from stagnation to develop and travel to the associated yang Organs. The bitter taste in the mouth and dry stools are also strong evidence that the lesser yang and yang brightness have been attacked.

2. What is the significance of the patient's pulse?

In this case the pulse is soft, but the right side is a little deeper. The soft pulse is typically floating, thin, and forceless, which is usually caused by poor circulation of qi and blood. The two most common causes of this pulse are invasion by dampness and a general deficiency of qi and blood. This patient, however, shows no evidence to suggest either of these patterns. Instead, here the pulse is due to wind obstructing the circulation of qi; there is no deficiency.

The pulse on the right side is a little deep, indicating that the pathogenic factors have penetrated to the interior of the body. The pulse on the right side is responsible for the following: Lung, Spleen, and Kidney yang. Palpating here allows us to assess the condition of the yang qi. In this case the pulse reveals obstruction of qi caused by the invasion of pathogenic factors and the resultant decrease in the movement of blood.

3. Is the patient's headache a symptom of a terminal yin pattern?

Headache at the vertex is generally regarded as a terminal yin disorder, but there are three channels which transverse the top of the head: the governing vessel, as well as the greater yang and lesser yang channels. This particular patient mainly complains of discomfort on the right side of the head; moreover there are other signs which point to yang brightness and lesser yang disorders. There is no evidence to suggest that the vertex symptom represents an independent pattern, and it is therefore not in the category of terminal yin headache.

4. How do you examine for facial paralysis?

When we examine patients with facial paralysis we want to precisely determine the affected site and also assess the extent of motor impairment. First, ask the patient to raise their eyebrows. This allows you to assess whether the wrinkles on the forehead have become shallow or have disappeared entirely. Second, ask the patient to close their eyes while you try to forcibly open them. This can help determine the strength of the orbicularis muscle. Third, visually examine the nasolabial folds to check if the affected side has either disappeared or merely become more shallow. Fourth, ask the patient to purse their lips, blow out their cheeks, and then show their teeth. If these movements cannot be carried out properly and the number of teeth revealed on one side is less than the other, the results are positive for a dysfunction of the orbicularis oris muscle. Fifth, check whether there is tenderness below the mastoid process, i.e., behind the ear.

If all the tests are positive then the diagnosis is peripheral facial paralysis, although in some cases tenderness may be absent from the mastoid process. If the facial paralysis is caused by a disorder of the central nervous system, then only the third and fourth tests will be positive, i.e., the symptoms affecting the nasolabial fold and mouth will be present, but the patient will be able to raise their eyebrows (because the central innervation of the forehead comes from both sides of the brain) and there will not be any tenderness around the mastoid process.

Conclusion

1. According to the eight principles:
   This is a combination of a channel-collateral and an interior pattern. There is heat and it is an excessive pattern.

2. According to etiology:
   Invasion by external pathogenic wind.

3. According to channels and collaterals:
   Heat from stagnation in the yang brightness and lesser yang channels (collateral pattern of windstroke).

4. According to Organ theory:
   Some heat from stagnation in the yang Organs.

Treatment principle

1. Expel the pathogenic wind and heat.
2. Remove the obstruction from the collaterals.

Selection of points

G-14 *(yang bai)* through to *yu yao* (M-HN-6) on right side
tai yang (M-HN-9) through to S-6 *(jia che)* on right side
S-3 *(ju liao)* through to LI-20 *(ying xiang)* on right side
S-4 *(di cang)* through to S-6 *(jia che)* on right side
qian zheng (N-HN-20) on right side
G-20 *(feng chi)*
LI-11 *(qu chi)*
TB-7 *(hui zong)*
G-8 *(shuai gu)*

Explanation of points

The local aspect of this treatment is four needles which stimulate seven points. These points and puncturing method are utilized in order to remove the obstruction from the collaterals and regulate the local circulation of qi and blood. Because the wind is in the superficial aspect of the body, this particular needling technique is employed. If a deep needling method were used, the pathogenic factors would only be driven deeper into the body. The yang brightness channel dominates this prescription, mainly because the yang brightness affects most areas of the face. Furthermore most patients dislike being needled on the face and threading reduces the number of needle punctures.

LI-11 *(qu chi)*: The principal function of this point is to clear heat. Stimulation of the point also leads to harmonization of the nutritive and protective levels, and subsequently to discharge of the wind from the collaterals.

G-20 *(feng chi)* is chosen to remove the wind, also to relieve the symptoms of exterior and channel-collateral patterns. There is a very close relationship between this point and problems of the head and eyes.

TB-7 *(hui zong)* is the accumulating point of the Triple Burner channel. Its principal function is to remove obstruction from the channel, promote local circulation, and alleviate pain.

G-8 *(shuai gu)* is mainly used for local channel problems. However it also has the ability to clear heat due to stagnation from the lesser yang channel.

qian zheng (N-HN-20) was found in clinical practice to have a good therapeutic effect on facial paralysis. The name of the point in Chinese means 'correct deviations.'

Combination of points

1. In this case, seven points on the face using four needles are combined collectively to affect the forehead, eye, cheek, nose, and mouth. Each pair can be used individually or combined with others to affect the designated area.

2. G-20 *(feng chi)* and TB-7 *(hui zong)*: These two points are from the lesser yang channels. Both are used to remove stagnation and promote circulation in the lesser yang channels, and thus alleviate pain.

Follow-up

The patient in this case was treated every day for six days with the same points. At this stage all of the symptoms had vanished except for a very slight deviation on the angle of the mouth when she smiled. The facial points were then only needled superficially (2-4mm) and there was no threading of the needles for four visits. This brought about a complete recovery.

Three days later she returned feeling unwell, although her facial disorder was completely gone. She complained of dizziness, heavy sensation in the head, pain in the right forehead, palpitations, shortness of breath, poor appetite, regurgitation, difficulty falling asleep, restlessness, nightmares, and dry mouth. The tongue was slightly dark red with a white, dry, and slightly thick coating. The pulse was sunken, thin, and slippery. This clearly indicated that the heat from stagnation in the lesser yang and yang brightness channels had disrupted the yang Organs and disturbed the spirit. New points were selected for treatment:

G-20 *(feng chi)*, rapid needling
LI-11 *(qu chi)*
H-7 *(shen men)*
GV-6 *(ji zhong)*

After two treatments the symptoms disappeared. The principles of treatment governing this selection of points were to clear heat from the yang Organs and calm the spirit. GV-6 *(ji zhong)* was drained here to clear heat from the middle burner.

CASE 30: **Female, age 52**

Main complaint

Numbness and motor impairment on the left side of the body

History

The patient's symptoms developed suddenly, and she came for treatment after just one day. On that day she had awakened with numbness down the left side of her face, arm, and leg. She also experienced frequent episodes of muscular weakness of the limbs. Each episode was of 2-3 minutes' duration.

The patient recalled that in the past she had experienced numbness on the tips of the fingers of the left hand, but she had ignored this and had never received treatment. Prior to her latest problem she caught a bad cold, and after a family dispute became angry and emotionally upset. At present, except for a stifling sensation in the chest, she has made a good recovery from her cold.

She had recently experienced other problems with her general health, including dizziness, restlessness, insomnia, dream-disturbed sleep, a feverish sensation on the upper half of her body, excessive sweating, dry throat, and thirst with a strong desire to drink. She reported that her lower back and limbs had felt weak, sore, and cold for a long time. The patient's blood pressure was normal. Her complexion was quite red, and her eyes were bloodshot.

Tongue

Dark red tongue with a white, greasy coating

Pulse

Right side is sunken and rapid, left side is sunken, thin, and rapid. Both pulses are forceless.

Analysis of symptoms

1. Numbness and motor impairment of the left side of the body—obstruction of the channels.

2. Dizziness—ascendant Liver yang.

3. Red complexion and eyes, feverish sensation on the upper aspect of the body, excessive sweating, dry throat, excessive thirst—heat in the upper burner.

4. Restlessness, insomnia, and dream-disturbed sleep—heat disturbing the spirit.

5. Weakness and soreness of the lower back and limbs—Kidney deficiency.

6. Coldness of the lower part of the body—yang deficiency in the lower burner.

7. Dark red tongue, rapid pulse—heat pattern.

8. Sunken, thin, forceless pulse—deficiency pattern.

Basic theory of case

An important concept in traditional Chinese medicine is that the Liver and Kidney share the same source of yin. They are both located in the lower burner. One of the physiological functions of the Liver is to store blood, while the Kidney stores vital essence. These functions are associated closely with the yin aspect of the body. There is a symbiotic relationship between the Liver blood and Kidney essence: the Kidney essence can be transformed into blood, and the blood nourishes the Kidney essence. They are thus interdependent for their mutual survival.

As a result of this close relationship, a disorder in one can easily upset the other. A typical example is known as *shuǐ bù hán mù* in Chinese. This means that the water phase cannot nourish and support the wood phase. The common cause of this pattern is Kidney yin deficiency leading to a pattern of Liver blood deficiency. This can eventually lead to both Liver blood and Liver yin deficiency. Similarly, Liver yin and blood deficiency can lead to Kidney yin deficiency. Because of the close relationship between the Liver and Kidney, a downward spiral of deteriorating health commonly occurs.

The yin and yang of the Liver coexist in a precarious harmony. When the yin of the Liver is deficient, the slightest spark is enough to cause ascendant Liver yang. When ascendant Liver yang becomes severe it will inevitably lead to internal wind.

Fig. 3

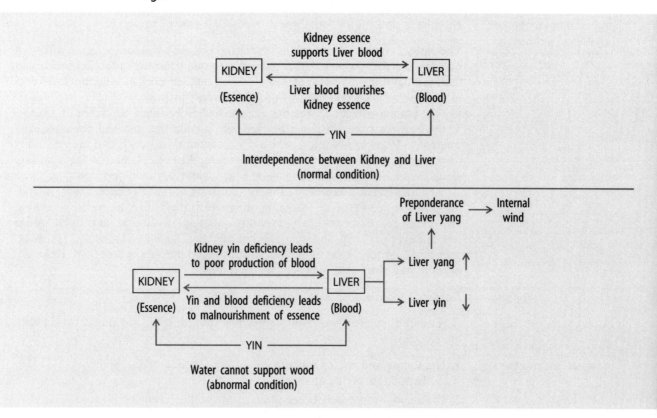

Interdependence between Kidney and Liver
(normal condition)

Water cannot support wood
(abnormal condition)

Cause of disease	1. Emotional change. 2. Deficiency of antipathogenic factor. Before the onset of the symptoms, the patient had a major emotional upset. This was the direct cause of her disorder. The patient also has a history of soreness and weakness on the lower parts of the body, and the pulse is sunken, thin, and forceless, indicating that she has a deficiency of antipathogenic factor.
Site of disease	Liver and Kidney A sudden onset of numbness and paralysis down one side of the body (here the left) is usually due to a Liver disorder, i.e., internal Liver wind. Soreness, weakness, and coldness in the lower back and lower limbs implies Kidney involvement.

Pathological change	The lower back is considered to be the dwelling of the Kidney, and the Liver is also situated in the lower burner. The blood and yin from the Liver and Kidney are essential for the nourishment of the lower burner, and therefore the symptoms will often begin to appear in this region before any other. This patient had problems in the lower back and lower limbs which existed long before the onset of her most recent disorder. This indicates a chronic deficiency of Liver and Kidney yin.
	    The heat from deficiency is caused by the yin deficiency. The heat pushes the qi and blood upwards to the head, thus the patient has a dry throat, thirst, red complexion, etc.. Moreover, the heat also disturbs the spirit which causes the patient's insomnia, restlessness, and dream-disturbed sleep.
	    The ability of the Liver to regulate the free-flowing of qi is closely related to the emotional state of the body. This patient had a history of emotional upset, and she still has a stifling sensation in the chest. This indicates stagnation of qi.

She also has a chronic imbalance of the Liver yin and yang. The yin deficiency is brought about by water failing to nourish wood. In these circumstances emotional upset will often give rise to severe ascendant Liver yang, i.e., Liver wind. The clear yang in the head is disrupted by the sudden upsurge of Liver wind. This explains why the patient experiences dizziness. The circulation of qi and blood in the head and channels is disrupted by the wind, and the patient therefore experiences numbness and paralysis down one side of the body. These symptoms are episodic because the wind is still very active; it could potentially develop further. This is the first day of onset of symptoms and the wind is in a very dangerous stage. If it continues to develop, a more typical hemiplegia will result.

The dark red tongue and rapid pulse indicate a disruption of the qi and blood by heat from deficiency. The thinness of the pulse on the left side, and the sunken, forceless nature of both pulses, indicates a deficiency of yin and blood.

Pure yin deficiency will exhibit only symptoms of heat, but in this case, besides the soreness and weakness of the lower back, the patient also feels cold, and the tongue coating is white and greasy. This indicates that the yang of the lower burner is also deficient, hence both the Kidney yin and yang are deficient.

Fig. 4

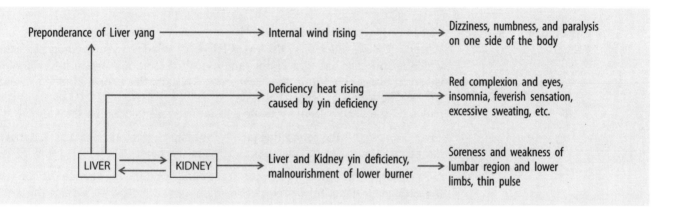

Pattern of disease

The onset of this patient's disorder is closely associated with her emotional upset. As mentioned earlier, the site of disease is the Liver and Kidney. There is no evidence of any exterior involvement; it is thus an interior pattern.

This case presents a combination of heat and cold, i.e., 'heat above with cold below'. The deficiency of yin creates heat from deficiency in the upper burner and head. The lower burner exhibits Kidney yang deficiency.

The root of this patient's disorder is deficiency of the Kidney and Liver, while the symptoms are those of internal wind. It is thus a pattern of deficiency.

Additional notes

1. Are there any external pathogenic factors in this case?

The cause of windstroke can be either external or internal wind. This patient had a bad cold before onset; did the wind also attack the collaterals and channels?

At present she has no symptoms of a bad cold, but she does display serious symptoms of Kidney and Liver deficiency. Obstruction of the channels and collaterals with major symptoms of heat from deficiency is evident, without any symptoms of external pathogenic wind. We therefore cannot say this patient has an exterior pattern.

2. Is it contradictory for there to be deficiency of both the yin and yang of the Kidney?

Because the yin and yang of the Kidney work very closely together, when one aspect becomes weak, the other will certainly follow. Thus simultaneous deficiency of Kidney yin and Kidney yang is not contradictory. In this case it is impossible to say which aspect became deficient first, which in any case is irrelevant. The real question is which of the two deficiencies should be corrected first.

Conclusion

1. According to the eight principles:
   Interior, heat above with cold below, deficiency.
2. According to etiology:
   Internal wind (Liver wind).
3. According to channels and collaterals:
   Windstroke, channel pattern.
4. According to Organ theory:
   Kidney and Liver yin deficiency leading to internal wind.
   Kidney yang deficiency.

Treatment principle

Nourish the yin, settle the yang, arrest the wind, clear the heat.

Selection of points

si shen cong (M-HN-1)	LI-6 *(pian li)*
TB-5 *(wai guan)*	Liv-5 *(li gou)*
L-7 *(lie que)*	K-4 *(da zhong)*
H-5 *(tong li)*	K-6 *(zhao hai)*

Explanation of points

si shen cong (M-HN-1): These points are located 1 unit posterior, anterior, and lateral to GV-20, which is on the top of the head. Wind is a yang pathogenic factor which in this case has attacked a yang aspect of the body. When internal wind is severe, disruption within the 'clear palace' results; this is also known as windstroke. The group of points known as *si shen cong* (M-HN-1) is situated on the crown of the head. Needling them arrests the wind and calms the spirit.

TB-5 *(wai guan)* is the connecting point of the hand lesser yang channel. It removes the obstruction from the channel and clears the heat.

L-7 *(lie que)* is the connecting point of the hand greater yang channel. It removes the pathogenic wind. In windstroke this point can help expel wind from the channels on the head.

H-5 *(tong li)* is the connecting point of the hand lesser yin channel. It nourishes the blood, calms the spirit, and arrests internal wind. It clears the obstruction from the hand lesser yin, and is a very useful point in treating both aphasia and dysphasia. It can also be used for stiffness of the tongue, dizziness, and vertigo.

LI-6 *(pian li)* is the connecting point of the hand yang brightness channel. This point can clear heat, especially from the upper burner.

Liv-5 *(li gou)* is the connecting point of the foot terminal yin channel. This point has an excellent ability to promote the free-flowing of Liver qi and is thus often used after windstroke to help restore the normal circulation of blood and qi.

K-4 *(da zhong)* is the connecting point of the foot lesser yin channel. It is a good point for promoting the activity of the Kidney, and thus alleviates many lower back symptoms.

K-6 *(zhao hai)* nourishes the yin of the Kidney and the whole body. It can also help calm the spirit and treat dryness of the throat.

Combination of points

H-5 *(tong li)* and K-6 *(zhao hai)* is a combination of upper and lower points on channels with the same name (here the lesser yin). It is an excellent combination for nourishing the yin and blood, and also for calming the spirit.

In this point prescription six connecting points are used, two from yang channels and four from yin channels. This is done in order to regulate the channels and promote the flow of qi.

Follow-up

After the first treatment the insomnia, restlessness, stifling sensation in the chest, and motor impairment virtually disappeared. The patient's mood became much more positive and optimistic. Two days later she received another treatment for episodic numbness. The points were changed to the following:

si shen cong (M-HN-1)
Connecting points of the six yang channels (yang brightness, lesser yang, and greater yang) were used on the left side of the body; connecting points of the six yin channels (terminal yin, lesser yin, and greater yin) were used on the right side.

This was done because of the relative laterality of yin and yang based on gender. In women the left side is usually considered the yin side, and the right the yang. In this case the internal wind occurred on the left (yin) side. To calm the wind and balance the yin and yang, the connecting points of the yang channels were used on the left, and those of the yin channels on the right. The patient responded well to treatment and the numbness disappeared immediately after treatment.

The patient returned two days later. This time the main complaint had become soreness of the muscles on the left side. The point selection was changed again to the connecting points of the yang brightness channel:

LI-6 *(pian li)*
S-40 *(feng long)*

After two treatments all the soreness was gone. The only remaining symptom was slight weakness of the lower back. The patient continued her treatment until this problem was resolved.

This woman had never before had acupuncture. She was very anxious about the degree of discomfort that she might experience, but all her friends and the medical personnel repeatedly recommended acupuncture to her. Such was the success of the treatment for her paralysis that she decided to continue her treatment until her back problem was resolved.

The selection of the connecting points can be quite specialized. Owing to their exterior-interior relationship, these points regulate the qi activity of both channels simultaneously. They are generally situated in very close proximity to one another, and thus the selection of which group to use is very important.

In this case, initially more connecting points from the yin channels were utilized to arrest the internal wind by nourishing the yin aspect of the body. Because the first treatment was successful, the objective of treatment then became one of balancing the yin and yang of the body. The yang connecting points were therefore used on the left side, and the yin connecting points on the right. The third treatment was changed in order to promote the function of the yang brightness channel alone, since the chief complaint had become soreness of the muscles.

CASE 31: **Female, age 39**

Main complaint

Unconsciousness and hemiplegia

History

This patient had a long history of severe hypertension with dizziness and headache. She was prescribed appropriate Western medication, but took it only occasionally.

Two days ago, while physically laboring, she suddenly lost consciousness and was admitted to hospital while still unconscious. Her eyes were tightly closed, her jaw was tightly clenched, and her breathing was very rough with a loud gurgling sound from the throat. She had severe hemiplegia down the left side of the body. Since the onset of symptoms she had no bowel movements. Her temperature was 38.8°C, her body was very hot to the touch, and her face was red.

Tongue	The tongue body is deep purple and curled up as a result of increased muscular tension, the coating is thick, greasy, dry, and yellow. (Note: Because the patient was unconscious and her jaw was clenched, a special mouth-gag was used to open the mouth.)
Pulse	Slippery, wiry, and forceful

Analysis of symptoms

1. Sudden loss of consciousness—severe disruption of the brain known in traditional Chinese medicine as 'misting of the clear palace', which refers to the brain.
2. Hemiplegia—obstruction of the channels.
3. Tightly closed eyes, clenched jaw, and rough breathing—
    obstruction of the yang qi.
4. Gurgling in the throat—phlegm.
5. Red complexion, hot body surface, constipation—heat pattern.
6. Curled tongue—obstruction of the channels.
7. Deep purplish tongue—heat pattern.
8. Dry, yellow, greasy tongue coating and slippery pulse—phlegm-heat.

Basic theory of case

According to the five phase theory the Liver is associated with wood, spring, and wind. In nature the wind is characterized by movement, while spring is associated with new development, growth, and rebirth.

The qualities of the Liver encompass both of these aspects. For example, it is said that the Liver controls the dispersal and free-flowing of qi *(gān zhǔ shū xiè)*. This includes regulation of the emotions, constant readjustment to the physiological rhythms of life, and the establishment of harmony between all the yin and yang Organs. Qi circulation is closely related to the circulation of blood. For this reason the regulation of the free-flow of qi by the Liver also serves to regulate the blood. In addition the Liver also has a close relationship with the transformation and transportation of food and water in the middle burner.

Cause of disease

1. Wind.
2. Phlegm-heat.

Wind is a yang pathogenic factor. Whenever wind attacks the body, the onset of disease will be very sudden and the symptoms will always involve movement, such as muscular spasms, trembling, convulsions, dizziness, etc. The severity and site of these symptoms may change very quickly. This patient's illness reflects a wind pattern.

The unconsciousness, gurgling in the throat, yellow and greasy tongue coating, and slippery pulse all clearly indicate the presence of phlegm-heat.

Site of disease

Heart and Liver

The loss of consciousness is the main indication of a Heart disorder.

The sudden onset of symptoms, hemiplegia, and wiry pulse indicate involvement of the Liver.

Pathological change

The patterns of internal and external wind share many characteristics. Both types of wind can have a sudden onset with changeable symptoms, and usually they attack the upper part of the body. Their origins, however, are completely different: external wind comes from the natural environment penetrating the defenses of the body through the skin; internal or Liver wind is created by an abrupt change of the yang qi of the body. There is thus no direct relationship between these two forms of wind.

This patient has a history of dizziness and headache which shows that she already had a preponderance of yang. Her present condition was caused by a sudden and dramatic rise of Liver wind. Wind combined with phlegm mists the 'clear palace' and disrupts the ascension of clear yang, leading to malnourishment of the head. The spirit therefore becomes incapable of maintaining consciousness.

As a result of Liver wind, the Liver's main activity of promoting the free-flow of qi is entirely disrupted, resulting in an imbalance between qi and blood, which causes severe stagnation. The yang qi is incapable of rising to the body surface, and thus cannot maintain the activity of the sensory organs. This explains why the patient has a tightly clenched jaw and tightly closed eyes. The hemiplegia is caused by obstruction of the channels and collaterals by wind and phlegm.

The circulation of Lung qi is interrupted by the phlegm-heat in the upper burner and consequently the patient has very rough breathing. The hot sensation of the body and the patient's red complexion are caused by the pathogenic heat rising upwards and bringing qi and blood with it. The patient is constipated not only because the general circulation of qi in the body has been thrown into chaos, but also because the pathogenic heat has consumed the fluids of the Large Intestine.

The tongue is deep purple due to pathogenic heat which has penetrated to the blood level. The curled tongue body indicates obstruction of the channels caused by internal wind and phlegm. The stiffness and immobility of the tongue are also symptoms of a more general pattern of channel obstruction causing malnourishment of the sinews, muscles, and vessels of the body. The dry, thick, yellow, and greasy tongue coating and slippery pulse are typical manifestations of phlegm-heat. The wiry nature of the pulse clearly indicates a Liver disorder.

Fig. 5

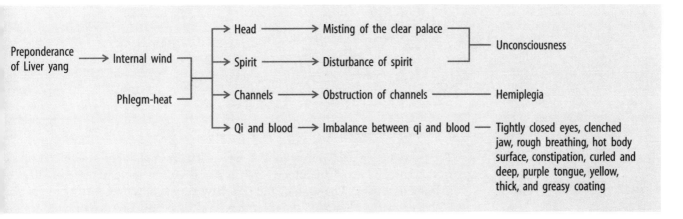

| Pattern of disease | Interior pattern: The internal wind was caused by an imbalance of yin and yang in the Liver which blocked the channels, misted the spirit, and interrupted the circulation of qi and blood.
Heat pattern: Red complexion, hot body surface, deep purple tongue, and yellow coating all confirm the presence of heat.
Excessive pattern: The main evidence for this is sudden unconsciousness, tightly closed eyes, clenched jaw, rough breathing, and wiry, slippery pulse. The great amount of phlegm has obstructed the flow of yang qi. |

Additional notes

1. Where did the phlegm come from?

There are two possible explanations. First, the patient has chronic Spleen qi deficiency. This pattern produces dampness, which can transform into phlegm if the condition persists for a long period of time. The second possibility is that the Liver wind could have caused chaos within the middle burner and induced the rapid production of phlegm.

Clinically however, phlegm, no matter where it originates, will manifest in the same way. The treatment principle will therefore be the same.

2. Is this case purely excessive?

Preponderance of Liver yang and the rising of Liver wind are both influenced by a deficiency of Kidney and Liver yin. These two individual patterns are therefore a combination of excess and deficiency. That is, the root of disease is deficiency, but the symptoms which characterize it are excessive.

According to the eight principles this should be classified under a deficiency heading (like case number 30), but in this case the pattern is described as excessive. The reason is that although yin deficiency is a problem, the combination of wind and phlegm-heat presents a strong set of pathogenic factors. They are all excessive in nature, which causes profound stagnation of qi. Therefore the symptoms of Kidney and Liver yin deficiency fade into insignificance, and the diagnosis focuses on excess as the main problem.

Fig. 6

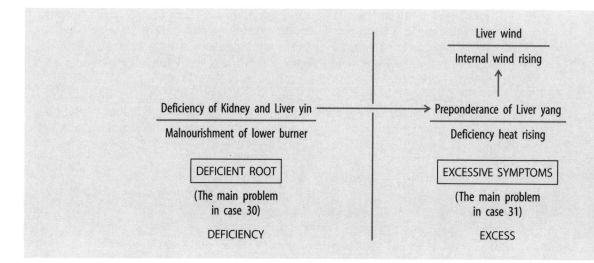

3. Is there blood stasis?

The patient has a deep purple tongue, which usually implies heat and blood stasis. In this case, however, the blood stasis is just a sign of the pathological changes that are occurring. The yang qi and heat have surged upwards, forcing the qi and blood upwards. They are all concentrated in the head where stagnation occurs. This phenomenon causes a collapse in circulation resulting in blood stasis.

4. Which pattern of windstroke is this?

The four key symptoms are: (i) unconsciousness, (ii) hemiplegia, (iii) tightly closed eyes, (iv) clenched jaw (also known as trismus). The yang qi is clearly very stagnant, hence this is part of the closed pattern of yang Organ windstroke.

Conclusion

1. According to the eight principles:
   Internal, heat, excessive pattern.

2. According to etiology:
   Internal wind (Liver wind), phlegm-heat.

3. According to Organ theory:
   Closed pattern of yang Organ windstroke.
   Liver wind with phlegm-heat misting the spirit.

Treatment principle

1. Calm the Liver, extinguish the wind.
2. Remove the phlegm and heat.
3. Open the orifices.

Selection of points	GV-26 *(ren zhong)* K-1 *(yong quan)* P-8 *(lao gong)* S-40 *(feng long)* Liv-3 *(tai chong)* 12 well points

Explanation of points

This point prescription is divided into two groups. The first five points are punctured with a strong reducing method. The 12 well points are bled, with the exception of K-1 *(yong quan)*.

GV-26 *(ren zhong)*: This point has a strong capacity to clear heat and recapture the spirit. Because the governing vessel is directly connected to the brain, the use of this point is indirectly instrumental in calming the Liver wind by improving the level of consciousness.

K-1 *(yong quan)*: This is the well point of the foot lesser yin channel. It has a good capacity to clear heat and remove obstruction from the brain and sensory organs, thus assisting in recapturing the spirit.

P-8 *(lao gong)*: This is the spring point of the hand terminal yin channel. It has a very strong effect on heat, which is disturbing the spirit. This point supports the function of GV-26 *(ren zhong)* and K-1 *(yong quan)*.

S-40 *(feng long)* is the connecting point of the foot yang brightness channel. It resolves phlegm and removes turbid yin (waste) from the body. Moreover, this point assists in regulating the flow of qi in the middle burner, thus helping to unblock the bowels.

Liv-3 *(tai chong)* calms Liver wind and clears heat, and is used here with a strong reducing method. It is a distant lower point and is a good combination with GV-26 *(ren zhong)*.

The second group of points are the 12 well points. The bleeding method is used to remove obstruction from the flow of qi and blood in the channels.

Combination of points

GV-26 *(ren zhong)*, K-1 *(yong quan)*, P-8 *(lao gong)*

These points clear the head and recapture the spirit. They are all located in very sensitive areas on the body, thus the needling sensation is very strong. Clinically, this combination is mainly used for the excessive pattern of unconsciousness. In addition, this combination includes one well point and one spring point which work together synergistically to reduce heat.

Follow-up

This patient was treated twice on the first day. Conventional emergency treatment was also given at the same time. After one day the tension in the patient was visibly reduced. The following day the patient was mentally clear, but the hemiplegia showed no signs of improvement. The treatment was then changed to one which mainly removed obstruction from the channels and collaterals. The points included:

GV-20 *(bai hui)*
LI-11 *(qu chi)*
TB-5 *(wai guan)*
G-34 *(yang ling quan)*
S-40 *(feng long)*
G-39 *(xuan zhong)*

After ten subsequent treatments the muscular strength started to recover. Two weeks later she could stand up with the support of a stick. Forty days after onset the patient could walk with a stick. After discharge from the hospital the patient continued to receive acupuncture treatment 2-3 times a week. Even though the rate of change slowed significantly after six months, she continued treatment for another eighteen months. During this time she was able to take care of herself and perform the activities of daily life. However, she still required a walking stick and her memory never recovered completely.

CASE 32: **Female, age 59**

Main complaint

Hemiplegia

History

The patient suffered a cerebral vascular accident (CVA) one month ago. At that time she suddenly lost consciousness and had obvious hemiplegia on the left side. After twenty-four hours in intensive care she regained consciousness.

She was first seen for acupuncture three weeks after the stroke. At that time her mental state was clear but she complained of weakness and numbness on the left side of the body and could not stand. There was deviation of the mouth to the right with salivation, and her speech was slurred. Her muscular strength was grade II to III. She felt that her tongue was very stiff. She had no appetite and no abnormal thirst. Her stools were dry with a bowel movement only once every several days.

Tongue

Dark with ecchymosis. The coating was thick, yellow, and greasy.

Pulse

Sunken, thin, and forceless

Analysis of symptoms

1. Unconsciousness and hemiplegia—windstroke.
2. Weakness and numbness of the limbs, deviation of the mouth, and slurred speech—obstruction in the channels and collaterals.
3. Loss of appetite—
   problem with transporting and transforming functions of the Spleen.
4. Dry stool and infrequent bowel movements—
   insufficient fluids in the Large Intestine.
5. Dark tongue with ecchymosis—blood stasis.
6. Thick, yellow, and greasy tongue coating—phlegm-heat.
7. Sunken, thin, and forceless pulse—deficiency.

Basic theory of case

In traditional Chinese medicine the qi and blood are closely related. In the first place, they mutually produce and transform into each other. They are also related in terms of circulation, and it is said that "Qi is the governor of the blood; blood is the mother of qi." This means that while the qi provides the energy for the movement of blood, it relies on the blood for its own production. It therefore follows that disorders of qi commonly result in blood stasis. There are two types of qi disorders that commonly lead to this situation in the clinic: qi stagnation leading to blood stasis, and qi deficiency leading to blood stasis.

i) Qi stagnation leading to blood stasis:

The qi stagnation occurs first, and this leads to poor blood circulation followed by stasis. Symptoms include localized pain with a distended or stifling sensation. There may also be a localized swelling or mass which is fixed, hard, and painful upon pressure. When the blood stasis is severe the patient may complain of sharp, stabbing pain. The tongue will be dark or have ecchymosis. The pulse is sunken and choppy.

ii) Qi deficiency leading to blood stasis:

Because of the deficiency of qi, there is a lack of energy to move the blood. The blood then slows down and stasis occurs. The patient will complain of fatigue or general lassitude, shortness of breath, and reluctance to speak. There may be a sharp, stabbing pain at various localized sites, which worsens with pressure. The tongue is pale with ecchymosis. The pulse will be sunken, choppy, and forceless.

The distinguishing characteristic between the two patterns is that in the case of qi stagnation the pattern is one of pure excess, whereas in qi deficiency there is a mixed picture of deficiency and excess. The treatment will therefore differ in each case.

Conversely, blood stasis can lead to qi stagnation. For example, factors such as cold or trauma can cause constriction or obstruction of the vessels. When this inevitably causes blood stasis, the qi will be prevented from moving and will also stagnate.

Cause of disease

1. Blood stasis.
2. Deficiency of antipathogenic factor.

The patient has suffered from hemiplegia for over one month and is unable to walk. This implies that there is poor circulation of qi and blood and obstruction of the channels and collaterals on one side of the body. The tongue is dark with ecchymosis, indicating blood stasis, which is the main cause of disease in this case.

The patient's appetite is poor and the pulse is sunken, thin, and forceless, indicating a deficiency of the antipathogenic factor.

Site of disease

Channels

The main evidence that the problem is in the channels is the fact that after one month the patient is still paralyzed and has difficulty in speaking.

Pathological change

Windstroke can be divided into three stages: acute, a period of recovery, and a chronic state with varying degrees of sequelae.

The acute stage may last from a few days to a few weeks. The patient's symptoms are very unstable, are at their most severe, and may change very rapidly. During the period of recovery the condition gradually stabilizes, depending on the treatment and the constitution of the patient. Varying degrees of recovery will occur. In the third stage the patient is left with some sequelae, and the rate of recovery becomes very slow or ceases.

There are obvious differences between the acute stage and that of recovery. In the acute stage there is rapid movement of internal wind and severe changes in the circulation of qi and blood. In addition the channels and possibly the head are obstructed by phlegm. In the stage of recovery the internal wind abates or disappears and obstruction in the channels becomes the main pathological change. Blood stasis is the most common cause at this stage. In addition, during the acute stage of this condition the rising Liver yang and Liver wind consume the body's yin. This leads to a severe imbalance between yin and yang which in turn depletes the antipathogenic factor. For this reason a deficiency of the antipathogenic factor is very common during the recovery as well as the chronic stage.

When this patient was in the first stage of windstroke, it was a yang Organ pattern. One month later the internal wind disturbance of qi and blood and obstruction of qi activity have improved, allowing the clear yang to go up to nourish the head. The disturbance of spirit has been relieved and the patient is conscious. However, hemiplegia, inability to walk, numbness, and slurred speech are still present. This indicates obstruction of the channels and malnourishment of the body.

When this case is compared with case number 31, the development of stroke can be seen very clearly. In the first stage, like case 31, the patient had sudden onset of unconsciousness, red complexion, hotness over the entire body, deep red tongue with yellow coating, evidence of the internal wind rising. Meanwhile, there was development of phlegm-heat with rough breathing, gurgling in the throat, thick and greasy tongue coating, and rolling and forceful pulse. Excessive pathogenic factor is obviously present. Unlike case 31, the patient's condition here is marked by deficiency of antipathogenic factors, including injury to the middle burner qi, Large Intestine qi, and body fluids. This is indicated by weakness of limbs and body, poor appetite, dry stools, and a sunken, thin, and forceless pulse. At the same time the dark tongue with ecchymosis indicates blood stasis. This case is thus a combination of deficiency and excess which has followed the first stage of internal wind and phlegm obstructing the channels. The deficiency here is that qi is consumed, and the excess appears as blood stasis.

Fig. 7

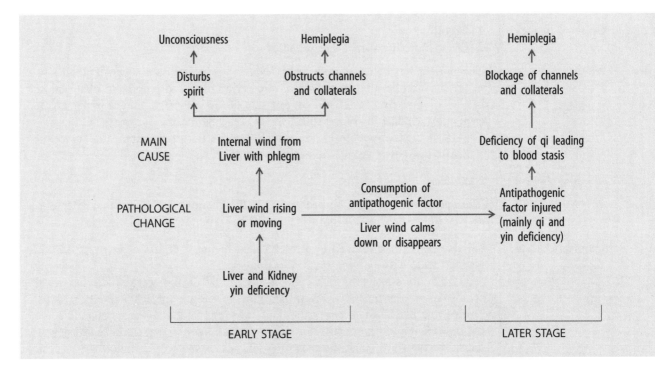

| Unconsciousness | Hemiplegia | | Hemiplegia |

| | | | |

Pattern of disease | This is an interior disorder because the patient's hemiplegia results from obstruction of qi and blood.

The pattern is one of heat because the stools are dry and the tongue coating is yellow and greasy.

There is a combination of deficiency and excess because, at this later stage of development of the stroke, the antipathogenic factor has been consumed, i.e. become deficient, and this deficiency of qi has led to blood stasis, an excessive condition.

Additional notes | 1. Is there phlegm present in this case?

Retention of phlegm is very common during the acute stage of windstroke. Although this patient has progressed to the stage of recovery, the tongue coating is still yellow, thick, and greasy which indicates phlegm-heat is still retained in the body. In this case, however, there are no other signs of phlegm-heat and is thus considered a minor factor that is merely a remnant of the acute stage.

2. Why is the patient constipated?

In this case there are two reasons: deficiency of qi, and injury to the body fluid.

by heat. The pathogenic heat is very strong during the acute stage and this causes the fluids in general to dry up, including those of the Large Intestine. At present the heat has almost disappeared but the body fluids have not fully recovered, and together with the qi deficiency, there is insufficient force to move the stool; thus the patient is constipated.

3. What is the cause of the hemiplegia at different stages of the windstroke?

Hemiplegia is the main symptom of windstroke. In traditional Chinese medicine the cause is regarded as wind and phlegm blocking the channels and collaterals, as in cases 30 and 31. It can also be caused by blood stasis in the channels and collaterals, as occurred in this case.

Phlegm is a substantial, turbid pathogenic factor which is yin in nature. It can move to a certain extent, but the speed and extent of movement is limited. Wind is invisible and transient and therefore yang in character, and can cause symptoms to appear very quickly in many different sites around the body. Wind seldom causes a fixed, permanent obstruction. In stroke patients there are always two internal pathogenic factors, wind and phlegm; the first is yang, moving, and invisible, the other yin, quiet, and visible. Wind and phlegm together can therefore sweep through the body causing widespread problems, blocking the channels in the head and body, and disturbing the spirit. This happens during the acute stage (see cases 30 and 31).

When windstroke develops to a later stage, the Liver wind calms down and the pathogenic wind-phlegm factor gradually becomes weaker or disappears. During the acute stage, however, the pathogenic factors are so strong that they injure the antipathogenic factor, and thereby weaken the qi of the body. The circulation of blood is impaired, leading to stasis; this is the main cause of hemiplegia as a sequelae to windstroke.

Conclusion	1. According to the eight principles: Interior, heat, and combined excess and deficiency pattern. 2. According to etiology: Blood stasis is the main cause, and there is also some residual phlegm-heat. 3. According to channels and collaterals: Windstroke (sequelae stage) and blood stasis in the channels. 4. According to qi, blood, and body fluids: Deficiency of qi causing blood stasis.
Treatment principle	1. Tonify the qi and remove the stagnation. 2. Regulate the qi in the channels.
Selection of points	S-36 *(zu san li)* Sp-10 *(xue hai)* G-20 *(feng chi)* CV-23 *(lian quan)* LI-11 *(qu chi)* S-40 *(feng long)*
Explanation of points	S-36 *(zu san li)* is an important point for tonifying the antipathogenic factor, and is also a local point for removing obstruction from the legs. Sp-10 *(xue hai)* has a strong action in regulating the blood and removing blood stasis. G-20 *(feng chi)* expels wind and removes obstruction from the channels in the head. CV-23 *(lian quan)* is close to the throat. It is used to clear the throat and remove heat and obstruction from the channels. It is particularly effective when the

patient has aphasia, and is also useful in removing phlegm.

LI-11 *(qu chi)* is used to clear heat from the entire body and remove obstruction from the upper limbs. It is an important point for treating paralysis and alleviating pain.

S-40 *(feng long)* is used to remove heat and clear phlegm. As a connecting point, it regulates the functions of the Stomach and Spleen channels.

Combination of points

S-36 *(zu san li)* and S-40 *(feng long)* tonify the qi and remove phlegm. Because they are located on the same channel, one point can be used on each side.

S-36 *(zu san li)* and Sp-10 *(xue hai)* tonify the qi and remove blood stasis.

G-20 *(feng chi)* and CV-23 *(lian quan)* are both located near the head. Together they clear obstruction from the entire head. Patients suffering from windstroke may have many symptoms affecting the head and face such as headache, dizziness, blurred vision, aphasia, and facial paralysis. These two points are thus very helpful, especially when the symptoms relate to the eyes, tongue and throat, or occiput.

Follow-up

This patient was treated three times weekly with basically the same set of points. After two weeks the muscular strength was obviously improved and salivation reduced. Her speech was also better. Four weeks later she was able to walk without assistance and to perform simple tasks such as dressing. The numbness on the left side of the body had disappeared. From this time she was treated only once or twice weekly, and although her treatment eventually became quite infrequent, she continued to improve. After six months of treatment there were no residual sequelae and treatment was suspended.

Diagnostic principles for windstroke

In Chinese the term for windstroke is *zhòng fēng*, meaning 'attacked by wind.' In traditional Chinese medicine windstroke includes two types of problems, one caused by invasion of external pathogenic wind, giving rise to an exterior pattern; the other caused by either external or internal wind which disturbs the qi and blood and gives rise to either an interior pattern or a channel-collateral pattern. Most cases involve an interior pattern only, and this discussion is mainly confined to that type.

Etiology and pathological change

The causes of windstroke are mainly pathogenic wind, phlegm, and blood stasis.

i) Wind

Wind includes external and internal wind. When the external wind attacks the surface of the body, it attacks the collaterals and disturbs the circulation of qi and blood. This is known as 'collateral-stroke' *(zhòng luò),* meaning that the collaterals have been attacked. This disorder is mild and localized.

Internal wind is caused by Liver and Kidney yin deficiency when ascendant Liver yang leads to internal wind. This disorder is usually widespread and the symptoms are severe. There are three types of stroke arising from internal wind: the channel type, yang Organ type, and yin Organ type. The internal wind rises, stirring up the qi and blood which then prevents the rising of the clear yang to the head, resulting in symptoms such as headache, dizziness, flushed face and restlessness, and causing problems in the channels pertaining to the head. This pure wind is regarded as disturbed qi, which will not cause long-term and severe obstruction of the channels.

ii) Phlegm

Phlegm is a pathogenic factor which is produced inside the body. There may be phlegm present in the body prior to a windstroke, or the internal wind may itself produce the phlegm. The circulation of qi is blocked, leading to poor circulation of blood. Phlegm combined with internal wind leads to severe obstruction in many parts of the body, including the channels and Organs.

iii) Blood stasis

This is the main pathogenic change in the late stage of windstroke. In the early stage when the wind and phlegm obstruct the channels, influencing the blood circulation, there are usually mild symptoms of blood stasis. After the acute stage the wind and phlegm gradually disappear and the blood stasis becomes more obvious; it is therefore at this late stage that blood stasis becomes the main pathogenic change.

In addition, there is a deficiency of antipathogenic factor during the onset and development of windstroke. In the early stage there is Kidney and Liver yin deficiency which causes internal wind. At a later stage the main problem is qi deficiency, which leads to blood stasis.

Fig. 8

Internal factors	Pathogenic factors	Site of disorder	Pathological change
Deficiency of antipathogenic factor and inability to check pathogenic factors	External wind ⟶	COLLATERALS ⟶	Obstruction of collaterals and malnourishment of superficial tissues
Liver and Kidney yin defiency, preponderance of Liver yang	Internal wind ⏐ Wind and phlegm ⟶ ⏐ Phlegm	CHANNELS AND ORGANS ⟶	Disturbance of qi and blood misting spirit
Chronic excessive phlegm or pathogenic water turns into phlegm			
Injury of antipathogenic factor and poor energy in circulating blood	Blood stagnation ⟶	CHANNELS AND COLLATERALS ⟶	Obstruction of channels and collaterals, poor circulation of blood

Types of windstroke

i) Collateral type

Numbness or paresthesia in the hands and feet, or mild motor impairment of a limb. There may be sudden weakness of the facial muscles on one side, leading to an inability to close the eye and deviation of the mouth. Salivation or mild speech problems may occur. The tongue coating is thin and white, and the pulse is wiry or floating.

ii) Channel type

The patient will initially suffer from headache, dizziness or tinnitus, soreness and weakness of the lower back and knee joints. There is then a sudden onset of facial weakness with deviation of the mouth and stiffness of the tongue with difficulty in speaking. There is also hemiplegia. The tongue is red with a yellow coating, and the pulse is wiry and thin or slippery and rapid.

iii) Yang Organ type

The patient has sudden loss of consciousness with clenched jaw, sonorous breathing, and spasms of the hand muscles. The patient seems hot and there is retention of urine and stool. Hemiplegia is also present. The tongue is red with a thick, yellow, greasy coating, and the pulse is sunken, slippery, rapid, and forceful.

iv) Yin Organ type

Sudden unconsciousness, the mouth is open, the breathing very weak, and the hand flaccid. The limbs feel cold and there is incontinence of urine and stool. The tongue is too weak to protrude, and the pulse is frail.

v) Sequelae type

There is hemiplegia with extreme weakness and sometimes numbness or paresthesia of the affected limbs. There is facial paralysis and usually some degree of aphasia. The complexion is sallow, the appetite is poor, the tongue is pale with ecchymosis, and the pulse is thin and choppy or weak and forceless.

In the clinical situation, one type may change or progress to another, becoming more or less severe as the case may be.

Diagnostic procedure for windstroke

The diagnosis mainly depends upon the pathogenic factors, the site of disease, and the strength of the antipathogenic factor.

Fig. 9

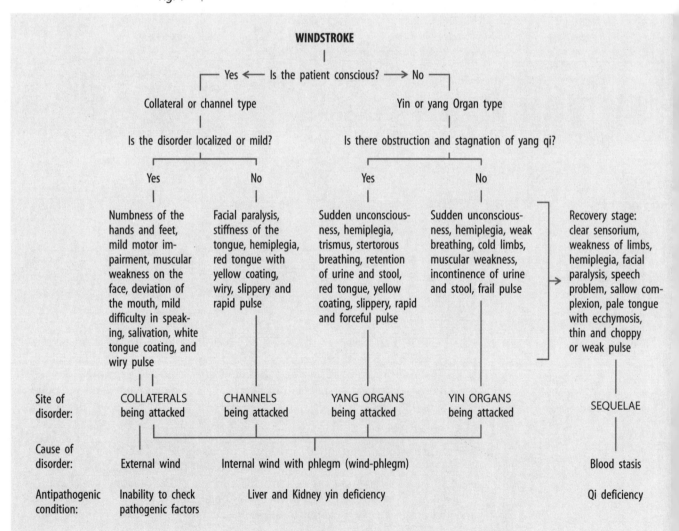

Insomnia

CASE 33: **Male, age 54**

Main complaint

Insomnia

History

One-year history of insomnia. The patient usually wakes between 3 and 4 A.M. and finds it difficult to fall back to sleep. He occasionally remembers his dreams. The patient feels that his level of mental energy during the day is poor, feels drowsy, and suffers from dizziness and poor memory. His food intake is less than average and he has abdominal distention after eating. He has general lassitude but is not restless and has no feelings of fever or cold. He is not thirsty. Urination and bowel movements are normal.

Tongue

Pale body with a thin white coating

Pulse

Thin

Analysis of symptoms

1. Early morning wakening and difficulty in falling back to sleep—malnourishment of the spirit.

2. Dizziness and poor memory—blood deficiency.

3. General lassitude, drowsiness, fatigue, reduced food intake, and abdominal distention—dysfunction of the Spleen.

4. Pale tongue and thin pulse—deficiency of qi and blood.

Basic theory of case

In the natural environment there is a constant succession of day following night, the day being governed by yang and the night by yin. In the individual there is a similar flow of energy, sleep being yin and wakening being yang.

During the day the yang qi is strong in the environment, and in the body the qi moves outwards to flow strongly in the yang channels. This energy keeps people alert and awake and enables them to carry out their normal daytime activities. When it begins to get dark the yang qi in the environment declines, and in the body the yang qi turns inwards, causing people to relax and become more quiet and less active. When the yang of the body completely enters the yin aspect the individual will fall asleep. Normal sleep is therefore controlled by two aspects, yin and yang, which must be balanced in order for yang to enter yin and conversely for yin to embrace yang. The Heart has the function of housing the spirit, and when it is peaceful the individual will sleep soundly.

Insomnia occurs when this coordination is lost and the spirit becomes disturbed.

Cause of disease	Deficiency of qi and blood

In this case there are no pathogenic factors. The patient is not restless and has no feeling of being either hot or cold.

The patient has insomnia, dizziness, poor memory, a pale tongue and a thin pulse, indicating deficiency of blood.

The general lassitude and fatigue with poor appetite and abdominal distention are symptoms of qi deficiency.

Site of disease   Heart and Spleen

Insomnia and poor memory are the main symptoms, which suggests a disorder of the Heart.

The poor appetite, abdominal distention, and general lassitude indicate involvement of the Spleen.

Pathological change   The Heart has two related functions, the first being to house the spirit, the second to control the blood vessels. A normal blood supply is the foundation on which a healthy spirit is built.

The function of the spirit includes thought processes and a normal sleep pattern. These are yang activities and they are supported by Heart blood, which is part of the yin of the Heart.

If there is deficiency of Heart blood the spirit will not be nourished and symptoms such as insomnia will occur. In Chinese medicine this pattern is called 'malnourishment of the heart and spirit' *(xīn shén shī yǎng)*. The typical patient will not have difficulty falling asleep, but will waken in the early hours and be unable to fall back to sleep. Generally speaking, they will not be restless and will dream very little. There may also be dizziness and poor memory because the spirit is deprived of blood.

There are many reasons for deficiency of Heart blood. In this case there are symptoms of poor appetite, abdominal distention, and general lassitude, indicating Spleen qi deficiency.

The Spleen has the function of transportation and transformation of food, and is regarded as the source of qi and blood. If there is Spleen qi deficiency this function will be lost and the food will not be transformed into vital essence, leading to lack of energy and a reduction in the generation of blood.

Fig. 1   The Spleen controls the muscles and limbs and malnourishment will occur if

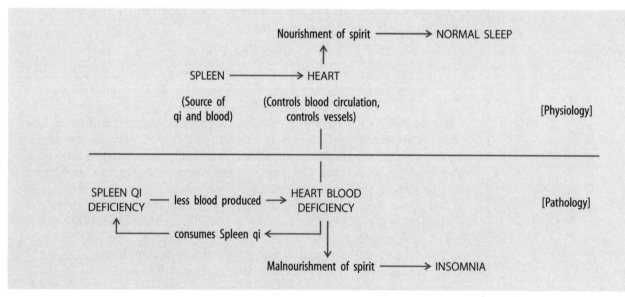

the Spleen qi is deficient, resulting in general lassitude and fatigue. The clear yang will be unable to rise and support the spirit, so there will be a lack of clarity of thought and the patient may feel drowsy. The Spleen also loses its ability to digest food, which then remains in the middle burner causing poor appetite and abdominal distention. *See Fig. 1.*

The tongue is pale because of blood deficiency and malnourishment. Because there is insufficient blood to fill the vessels, the pulse becomes weak and thin. The patient is not restless, feverish, or thirsty, so there is no evidence of heat. Neither is cold involved since there is no aversion to cold and the patient does not feel cold.

Pattern of disease

In this case there is no history of invasion by pathogenic factors. The main complaint is insomnia and the Heart and Spleen are involved. This pattern is interior.

All the symptoms involve qi and blood deficiency; there is a preponderance of neither yin nor yang, and there is thus no heat or cold.

The qi and blood are both deficient so this pattern is of course one of deficiency.

Additional notes

Which takes priority in this case, the Spleen qi deficiency or the Heart blood deficiency?

Qi and blood theory includes the concept that qi and blood depend on each other and transform into each other. Spleen qi deficiency leads to disruption in the transportation and transformation of food, and the long-term result will be blood deficiency. On the other hand, blood is a substantial material within the body which normally supports the qi, so that if there is blood loss for any reason the inevitable consequence will be qi deficiency. Qi and blood are mutually dependent, and deficiency of both is common in the clinical situation. In this case the symptoms involve deficiency of qi and blood, but the history does not reveal which is primary. Spleen qi deficiency may take priority in this case, but it is of no importance because it will not influence the treatment principle.

Conclusion

1. According to the eight principles:
   Interior, neither heat nor cold, and deficiency pattern.

2. According to Organ theory:
   Deficiency of Heart blood and Spleen qi. (In Chinese medicine this combination is always referred to as deficiency of the Heart and Spleen, and this will be the term used elsewhere in this book).

Treatment principle

1. Tonify the Spleen qi.
2. Nourish the Heart blood.
3. Calm the spirit.

Selection of points

S-36 *(zu san li)*
CV-12 *(zhong wan)*
H-7 *(shen men)*
Sp-6 *(san yin jiao)*

Explanation of points

S-36 *(zu san li)* is one of the most important tonifying points. It especially strengthens the middle burner qi and also the yang of the body to improve the general condition. It is therefore a good point to use in treating patterns of deficiency, or when the patient has a weak constitution.

CV-12 *(zhong wan)* is the alarm point of the Stomach on the conception vessel and is located in the middle burner. It is a good choice for regulating the middle burner and is commonly used for this type of disorder.

H-7 *(shen men)* is the source point of the Heart channel and is a good choice for calming the spirit.

Sp-6 *(san yin jiao)* is the meeting point of the three yin foot channels and has the general effect of nourishing the yin of the body, including the blood, vital essence, and body fluids.

Combination of points

S-36 *(zu san li)*, CV-12 *(zhong wan)*

One point is a local point and one distant for the middle burner; the pair thus involves both tonifying and regulating the qi or yang of the middle burner. In Chinese medicine the distant point is always more powerful than the local, so they are most effective when used in combination.

H-7 *(shen men)*, Sp-6 *(san yin jiao)*

This is the most common formula for insomnia. H-7 *(shen men)* calms the spirit while Sp-6 *(san yin jiao)* nourishes the yin, thus the balance between yin and yang is reestablished.

Follow-up

This patient received six treatments over three weeks after which he was sleeping for an additional 2-3 hours every night. His energy was improved and his spirit was clear. He had less abdominal distention. After two more weeks of two treatments per week he was sleeping well and only occasionally woke early in the morning. He had a good appetite and no abdominal distention. There was no long-term follow-up of this patient.

CASE 34: **Female, age 32**

Main complaint

Insomnia

History

Two months ago this patient was studying hard, with considerable mental strain, and began to suffer from insomnia. She had great difficulty in falling asleep and tossed and turned in bed. When she did sleep she dreamed a lot and had a tendency to wake with a start during a dream. Her memory became poor.

She also suffered from palpitations, restlessness, shortness of breath, and was reluctant to speak to anyone. She had night sweats, general lassitude, and her appetite was sometimes poor and sometimes normal. Bowel movement and urination were normal. Her menstrual cycle was regular, but the quantity of blood loss was reduced.

Tongue

Red at the tip, thin, yellow, greasy coating

Pulse

Wiry, thin, and rapid

Analysis of symptoms

1. Difficulty in falling asleep with many dreams and sudden wakening—
   spirit disturbed by heat.
2. Restlessness, palpitations, and night sweats—
   internal heat caused by yin deficiency.
3. Poor memory—malnourishment of the spirit.
4. Shortness of breath, poor appetite, and general lassitude—
   Spleen qi deficiency.
5. Reduced menstrual blood—blood deficiency.
6. Redness of the tongue tip, yellow tongue coating, and rapid pulse—heat.
7. Thin pulse—blood deficiency.

Basic theory of case

Insomnia is the general term for sleep disorders. In fact, in clinical practice there are several different types:

i. Difficulty in falling asleep means that insomnia occurs during the first stage of sleep irrespective of whether the patient goes to bed early or late. Sometimes the individual will eventually fall asleep after 1-2 hours of restlessness, and this leads to a vicious circle of anxiety about falling asleep and insomnia.

ii. Early wakening after which the patient cannot fall back to sleep, occurring in the late stage of sleep. There is no initial difficulty in falling asleep when the patient goes to bed. Most patients are not restless.

iii. Some people complain of a generally poor quality of sleep. They fall asleep easily but do not sleep deeply and may waken several times during the night. Their sleep is often disturbed by dreams. This type of disturbance affects the whole sleep pattern and the individual does not feel refreshed after a night's rest.

iv. Occasionally a patient will be unable to sleep at all during the entire night, but this is uncommon.

Insomnia is thus a complicated problem with many different symptoms which are of varying clinical significance. A careful history is therefore essential.

Cause of disease

1. Pathogenic heat.
2. Deficiency of qi and blood.

In this case the characteristics of insomnia are difficulty in falling asleep with restlessness, dream-disturbed sleep, and sudden wakening. These symptoms indicate that pathogenic heat is disturbing the spirit.

The poor memory and reduced menstrual flow are symptoms of blood deficiency.

Shortness of breath, general lassitude, and a reluctance to talk are signs of qi deficiency.

Site of disease

Heart and Spleen

Insomnia, palpitations, restlessness, and poor memory indicate that the Heart is affected.

Shortness of breath, general lassitude, and poor appetite are caused by a disorder of the Spleen.

Pathological change

The Heart houses the spirit which functions properly only when it is well-nourished by Heart blood and yin. Mental strain consumes both Heart yin and Heart blood and this leads to insomnia.

Blood pertains to yin but is not the same as yin, so the symptoms caused by blood deficiency and yin deficiency together are different from those of blood deficiency alone. Yin deficiency leads to internal heat which rises to disturb the spirit, causing difficulty in falling asleep, tossing and turning, with a lot of dreams and sudden wakening. Yin and blood deficiency leads to malnourishment of the spirit, which affects the memory. The heat caused by yin deficiency disturbs the Heart, resulting in palpitations and restlessness, and the heat has a tendency to push out body fluids through the pores in the form of sweat. This occurs especially at night when the deficient yin is unable to fully embrace the yang.

Mental strain also injures the Spleen. Under normal circumstances if someone studies very hard or thinks constantly about a problem, their appetite is often affected. This patient has a history of mental strain; the Spleen qi has thus been injured, especially in respect to its function of transportation and transformation. This resulted in poor appetite, general lassitude, and shortness of breath.

Because there is both yin and blood deficiency, the penetrating vessel, which is considered to be the 'sea of blood', has lost nourishment, leading to reduced menstrual bleeding.

Fig. 2

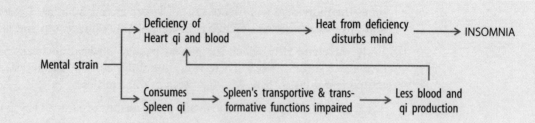

Pattern of disease

The tip of the tongue relates to the Heart, thus Heart yin deficiency is reflected in the red color which indicates heat or fire. The yellow tongue coating is also a sign of heat.

Blood deficiency results in a reduction of blood circulating to fill the vessels, thus the pulse is thin, but also rapid, because of the presence of heat.

There is no invasion by external pathogenic factors. The patient has a history of mental strain which has injured the Heart; it is thus an interior pattern.

There is restlessness, night sweats, a red tongue with yellow coating, and a rapid pulse indicating a heat pattern.

The characteristics of the insomnia accompanied by general lassitude, shortness of breath, reduced menstruation, and thin pulse are all part of a pattern of deficiency.

Additional notes

1. How does one distinguish insomnia caused by blood deficiency from insomnia caused by yin deficiency?

Blood deficiency causes insomnia characterized by early wakening with difficulty in falling back to sleep, but without restlessness or dreaming. Yin deficiency results in difficulty in falling asleep, dream-disturbed sleep, restlessness, and even irritability.

2. Is there deficiency of Lung qi in this case?

The Lung controls the qi of the entire body and Lung qi is responsible for the larynx and hence the voice. Where there is Lung qi deficiency the energy is reduced in the larynx and the patient will have a weak voice and be reluctant to speak. This patient has Spleen qi deficiency leading to reduced production of qi, so the Lung is not supplied with sufficient energy by the Spleen. The Lung disorder is therefore secondary to the disorder in the Spleen, and there are no other symptoms directly involving the Lung in this case. The diagnosis of Lung qi deficiency is therefore inappropriate.

3. Is the Liver involved in this case?

The Liver stores the blood and controls the volume of blood in circulation at any given time. In the case of Liver blood deficiency in women, the menstrual bleeding is reduced. This patient also has a wiry pulse which is commonly seen in disorders of the Liver and Gallbladder. In this case, however, the primary problem lies in the deficiency of Heart blood and yin, which can in turn affect the blood-storing function of the Liver. The symptoms relating to the Liver are therefore of secondary importance. In the absence of the cardinal signs and symptoms of Liver blood deficiency such as dizziness, pale complexion, poor night vision, or dry fingernails there is no reason to make that diagnosis.

4. Why is the tongue coating greasy?

A greasy tongue coating always implies dampness or phlegm. In this case the coating is also yellow, so there is some damp-heat present. The patient has Spleen qi deficiency, so in addition to poor appetite she also has a problem with water metabolism and there is some accumulation of dampness. The heat caused by the yin deficiency combines with this dampness to produce damp-heat. The coating is quite thin, indicating that the damp-heat is not particularly severe and has not given rise to other symptoms. When the Spleen recovers its normal function, this degree of dampness will resolve naturally.

Conclusion

1. According to the eight principles:
   Interior, heat, and deficiency pattern.

2. According to Organ theory:
   Heart blood and yin deficiency.
   Spleen qi deficiency.

Treatment principle

1. Clear the heat and calm the spirit.
2. Nourish the yin and blood.
3. Tonify the Spleen qi.

Selection of points

H-6 *(yin xi)*
GV-13 *(tao dao)*
K-7 *(fu liu)*
TB-5 *(wai guan)* through to P-6 *(nei guan)*

Explanation of points

H-6 *(yin xi)* has the function of removing heat caused by yin deficiency and calming the spirit. It is the accumulating point of the Heart channel.

GV-13 *(tao dao)* is the meeting point of the foot greater yang channel and the governing vessel. This is a very good point for removing internal heat caused by yin deficiency.

K-7 *(fu liu)* is an important point for the treatment of excessive sweating, including both spontaneous sweating and night sweats. It also clears heat.

TB-5 *(wai guan)* through to P-6 *(nei guan)*: Because both of these points are connecting points they are used to regulate the yin and yang between these two channels. P-6 *(nei guan)* has the function of calming the spirit and its main effect is on the upper and middle burners. TB-5 *(wai guan)* promotes the function of the Triple Burner to help calm the spirit. It particularly strengthens the middle burner.

In this selection there are no points which directly tonify the Spleen qi because this is a long-term problem which can be addressed when the insomnia begins to improve. P-6 *(nei guan)* does not tonify the qi, but it does have the function of regulating the qi in the middle and upper burners, thus helping the middle burner to recover normal function.

Combination of points

H-6 *(yin xi)*, GV-13 *(tao dao)*, K-7 *(fu liu)*: This is a small formula to clear heat caused by yin deficiency, especially when there are night sweats and insomnia.

Follow-up

This patient received three treatments during the first week, after which she dreamed very little but still had difficulty in falling asleep. After two more weeks of treatments every other day her sleep pattern became very stable and her menstrual flow returned to normal in the following cycle. Because her energy was also normal, no further treatment was given.

CASE 35: **Male, age 39**

Main complaint

Insomnia

History | This patient has suffered from recurrent insomnia for several years. During the past week the insomnia has returned with difficulty in falling asleep and many dreams. The patient usually feels restless and has a sensation of heat in the chest. He also suffers from dizziness, poor memory, and a weak appetite. His mouth is dry and he likes to drink water. He has slight soreness and weakness in the lower back and the knee joints. Bowel movement and urination are normal.

Tongue | Light red body with a thin yellow coating

Pulse | Sunken, thin, and slightly rapid

Analysis of symptoms |

1. Difficulty in falling asleep with many dreams—heat disturbing the spirit.

2. Restlessness, dizziness, poor memory, and dryness in the mouth— yin deficiency leading to internal heat.

3. Soreness and weakness of the lower back and knee joints— Kidney yin deficiency.

4. Yellow tongue coating and rapid pulse—heat.

5. Thin pulse—deficiency.

Basic theory of case | The Heart is located in the upper burner and is considered to be yang; the Kidney is in the lower burner and is considered to be yin. According to five phase theory, the Heart pertains to fire and the Kidney to water, and they are closely related.

Under normal conditions the Heart fire descends to the Kidney, where it helps Kidney yang to warm the Kidney yin which in turn nourishes the Organs. The Kidney water is therefore not too cold, and this water ascends to the Heart where it nourishes the Heart yin in preventing the Heart yang or fire from becoming too strong. In Chinese medicine this relationship is known as harmony between

Fig. 3 | the Heart and Kidney, or harmony between fire and water.

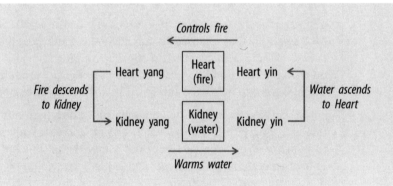

Cause of disease |

1. Heat.
2. Deficiency of yin.

The patient has insomnia characterized by difficulty in falling asleep and much dreaming. He also has a dry mouth and feels restless, indicating the presence of heat.

There are also several symptoms of internal heat, together with soreness and weakness of the lower back. The tongue coating is yellow and the pulse is sunken, thin, and rapid. All of these symptoms indicate yin deficiency.

Site of disease | Heart and Kidney

The patient has insomnia, a restless feeling in the chest, and poor memory, all of which involve the Heart.

Soreness and weakness of the lower back and knee joints are evidence of a Kidney disorder.

Pathological change

When the normal physiological relationship between the Heart and Kidney is broken there will be disharmony between the Heart yang and the Kidney yin. The initial reason may lie in either the Heart or the Kidney. If initially there is a preponderance of Heart fire the heat will descend and consume the Kidney yin or water, which in turn will be unable to control the Heart fire, and this cycle will continue. On the other hand, Kidney yin deficiency leads to Heart yin deficiency and hence to a preponderance of Heart fire.

Fig. 4

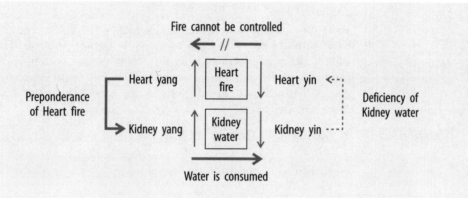

The patient has a history of insomnia for several years, thus the antipathogenic factors have been injured. There is yin deficiency leading to a relative excess of yang. This heat from deficiency, or 'empty' heat, has disturbed the spirit, thus the patient finds it difficult to fall asleep, dreams a lot, and is restless with a hot feeling in the chest. The deficiency of yin means that the spirit loses its normal nourishment and the memory weakens.

The lower back is the 'dwelling of the Kidney', and the Kidney controls bone and marrow. Kidney yin deficiency leads to malnourishment of the lower back and knee joints, resulting in soreness and weakness.

There are two possible reasons for the dizziness. Heart yin deficiency means that the spirit is undernourished, leading to dizziness. Or the deficiency of Kidney yin may cause the 'sea of marrow' or brain to become impoverished, which may likewise result in dizziness.

The dryness in the mouth can be explained by the yin deficiency and preponderance of fire. Because of the internal heat the patient has a yellow tongue coating and a rapid pulse. Heat tends to consume the body fluids, which are also reduced as part of the general yin deficiency, so the blood vessels will not be adequately filled and the pulse becomes thin.

Pattern of disease

The history is long and involves the Organs, and there is no invasion by external pathogenic factors; it is thus an interior pattern.

The patient is restless with a dry mouth, yellow tongue coating, and rapid pulse indicating a pattern of heat.

There is deficiency of yin, thus it is also a pattern of deficiency.

Additional notes

1. Why is there no excessive heat in this case?

Insomnia can be caused by heat disturbing the spirit, which can be either due to an excess of heat itself or to heat from deficiency (also known as 'empty heat') caused by a deficiency of yin and hence a relative preponderance of yang. There are no symptoms of invasion of the Organs by external pathogenic heat or of hyperactivity of yang, so this heat is entirely from deficiency.

2. In cases of insomnia, how does one distinguish Heart and Kidney disharmony from deficiency of Heart yin?

It is important to take a careful history in cases of insomnia so that symptoms of Kidney yin deficiency will not be missed, as Heart yin deficiency can occur without involvement of the Kidney. The symptoms of insomnia will be identical, but in the case of disharmony between the Heart and Kidney there will always be lower back pain, soreness and weakness of the lower limbs or knees, or nocturnal seminal emission with dream-disturbed sleep.

3. Why is there poor appetite?

Poor appetite is always related to disorder of the Spleen and Stomach, but in this case there are no other signs of a middle burner problem. The poor appetite is of secondary importance, is by no means the main complaint, and is probably the result of the long-term insomnia which has undermined the patient's general energy. Thus the poor appetite in this case is not evidence of any significant middle burner qi deficiency.

Conclusion	1. According to the eight principles: Interior, heat, and deficient. 2. According to yin-yang theory: Yin deficiency. 3. According to Organ theory: Disharmony between the Heart and Kidney.
Treatment principle	1. Harmonize the Heart and Kidney. 2. Nourish the yin, clear the heat, and calm the spirit.
Selection of points	GV-20 *(bai hui)* H-7 *(shen men)* Sp-6 *(san yin jiao)* S-38 *(tiao kou)* through to B-57 *(cheng shan)*

Explanation of points

GV-20 *(bai hui)* can be used to calm the spirit irrespective of the source of its disturbance, e.g., heat, wind, phlegm, or preponderance of yang.

H-7 *(shen men)* functions well in clearing the heat and calming the spirit by removing obstruction from the Heart channel.

Sp-6 *(san yin jiao)* is used to nourish the Kidney yin as it is the meeting point of the three foot yin channels. It is also useful for nourishing the blood and thus improving the function of the spirit.

S-38 *(tiao kou)* through to B-57 *(cheng shan)*: This point is more commonly used to treat acute shoulder problems, but here it serves a different purpose. S-38 *(tiao kou)* is a point on the foot yang brightness channel which is especially rich in qi and blood; it is therefore a good selection for removing heat and dampness. By puncturing through to B-57 *(cheng shan)* the heat is drained from yang brightness to greater yang and excreted via the Bladder channel. The greater yang channel is interiorly / exteriorly related to the Kidney channel, thus Kidney function will tend to improve when this point combination is used.

Follow-up

The insomnia disappeared after one treatment, and because the patient was very busy he did not return. In fact he should have undergone a full course of treatment, as his insomnia recurred whenever he encountered increased stress. He would then come back for one or two treatments which would cure the insomnia temporarily. This was not a satisfactory solution, but it suited this particular patient.

CASE 36: **Male, age 39**

Main complaint

Insomnia

History

Frequent insomnia for the past two years. It is not difficult to fall asleep initially, but he has many dreams and wakens easily, after which he finds it difficult to go back to sleep. The patient feels very restless and sometimes has a hot, feverish sensation with sweating when the restlessness becomes severe. In addition, he sometimes wakes up to find that he has been sweating during sleep. In Chinese medicine this is referred to as 'night sweats'. The patient has dizziness in the morning with a heavy sensation around the head, and high frequency, 'cicada-like' tinnitus. He also complains of poor memory, severe general lassitude, and feels cold all the time, with cold extremities. He is very sensitive to temperature changes and has an aversion to heat and cold alike, being unable to adapt quickly. His appetite is poor and he has very bad digestion. He has a dry mouth, likes to drink water, and complains of urinary frequency, getting up 3-4 times a night to urinate. He has loose stools with a bowel movement once per day. He also complains of pain and coldness of the knee joints. His complexion is pale.

Tongue

Dark red body with a yellow, dry, greasy coating, thick in the middle and at the root

Pulse

Right side: Slippery and forceless. The proximal position is thin.
Left side: Sunken, slippery, and forceless.

The distal position on each side is very weak, the left being weaker than the right.

Analysis of symptoms

1. Insomnia and dream-disturbed sleep with a tendency to wake easily and then have difficulty falling back to sleep—disturbed spirit.
2. Restlessness, night sweats, dryness of the mouth, and tinnitus—heat from yin deficiency.
3. Poor memory—malnourished spirit.
4. Feeling of cold and cold extremities—internal cold from yang deficiency.
5. Poor appetite, bad digestion, and loose stools—Spleen yang deficiency.
6. Cold and painful knee joints, urinary frequency, and nocturia—Kidney deficiency.
7. Dark red tongue with yellow coating, slippery pulse—heat.
8. Pale complexion, forceless pulse—cold from yang deficiency.

Basic theory of case

In the study of Chinese medicine one of the most fundamental distinctions which must be made is between patterns of heat and cold. A heat pattern manifests when there is either a preponderance of yang or deficiency of yin, while a cold pattern results when there is a deficiency of yang or preponderance of yin. In fact, patterns of heat and cold reflect an imbalance between yin and yang.

The patient manifesting a cold pattern will express feelings of being cold, and have cold extremities and a pale complexion. There is an absence of thirst and the stools will be loose or watery. The tongue is pale with a white coating and the pulse is slow.

A pattern of heat is present when the patient feels hot and expresses a preference for coolness, is thirsty, has a red complexion, and is constipated. The tongue is red with a yellow coating and the pulse is rapid.

These patterns of heat and cold are at opposite ends of the spectrum, but in an individual patient they may often occur together. In Chinese diagnosis this condition is known as a heat and cold complex. There are four main types which occur in clinical practice:

i. Exterior cold and interior heat

The patient has an exterior cold pattern with an aversion to cold, fever without sweating, and general aching. At the same time there is interior heat with restlessness, thirst, cough with thick, yellow sputum, a red tongue, and a rapid pulse.

ii. Exterior heat and interior cold

An exterior heat pattern exists when the patient has been exposed to wind-heat and at the same time has yang deficiency. The manifestations may include, e.g., fever with slight aversion to wind and cold, slight sweating, and a sore throat. There can also be abdominal pain which is relieved with warmth and pressure. The patient is afraid to take cold food and drink, the stools are loose or watery, the tongue is pale with a white coating, and the pulse is thin and forceless.

iii. Cold above and heat below

The cold pattern here is mainly in the upper part of the body, and the heat primarily affects the lower part. For example, the patient may have cold in the Stomach and damp-heat in the Bladder. The symptoms will be coldness and pain in the epigastric region, which is aggravated by cold, and vomiting of clear fluid. At the same time there will be frequency, urgency, and scalding pain when urinating, and the urine will be yellow. The tongue will be pale, but with a yellow, greasy coating, and the pulse is thin and forceless.

iv. Heat above and cold below

The heat pattern is in the upper part of the body, and the cold is lower down. For example, the heat may be in the Lung while there is cold from deficiency in the middle burner. There will be cough or asthma with thick, yellow, sticky sputum and at the same time the patient will have coldness and pain in the abdomen with poor appetite and loose or watery stools. The tongue coating will be yellow and greasy, and the pulse slippery, thin, and forceless.

It is important to judge both the location of the heat and cold and also the relative severity of each pattern.

Cause of disease

1. Heat.
2. Deficiency of yang.

This patient has insomnia with dream-disturbed sleep and difficulty in falling back to sleep if he wakes. He is restless and sometimes sweats, has a dry mouth, and high-frequency tinnitus. These symptoms all indicate that the spirit is disturbed by heat.

The patient always feels cold and has cold extremities, general lassitude, and loose stools, showing yang deficiency.

Site of disease

Heart, Spleen, and Kidney

Insomnia, restlessness, and poor memory are the main symptoms indicating that the Heart is involved.

The poor appetite, loose stools, and general lassitude are signs that there is dysfunction of the Spleen.

Frequent urination, nocturia, and pain and coldness of the knees indicate a Kidney disorder.

Pathological change

This case is a combination of heat and cold patterns. There is heat in the Heart and cold in the Spleen and Kidney; it is thus a pattern of heat above with cold below.

There are two causes for the insomnia in this case. First, the patient does not have difficulty in falling asleep but wakens early. This is characteristic of Heart blood deficiency leading to malnourishment of the spirit. In addition, he has dream-disturbed sleep and restlessness during the night, sometimes with sweating. This type of insomnia is caused by heat from deficiency, or 'empty heat', due to yin deficiency. The heat disturbs the spirit and prevents sleep. The pattern is therefore a mixture of Heart blood and Heart yin deficiency.

During the night the yin deficiency means that the yin cannot embrace the yang, and there is a preponderance of yang or 'empty heat.' This in turn causes some of the body fluids to convert to steam, which is then pushed out through the pores, causing night sweats.

The tinnitus is caused by the heat rising to disturb the ears. The poor memory is caused by malnourishment of the spirit resulting from both Heart blood and Heart yin deficiency. The patient has a dry mouth and is thirsty because heat consumes the body fluids. The above symptoms all involve the Heart, and heat is the main characteristic.

There is also Spleen qi deficiency with dysfunction of the Spleen in transporting and transforming food. The patient therefore has a poor appetite and bad digestion. There is an inability to extract sufficient vital essence from the food, which translates into severe general lassitude. The loose stools are typical of Spleen qi deficiency. There is dizziness with a heavy sensation round the head which indicates that the clear yang, which is part of Spleen qi, cannot rise to the head.

The Kidney is one of the main Organs that regulates water metabolism. It also controls the functioning of the Bladder. Kidney yang deficiency results in failure to warm and also to reabsorb water, so there is urinary frequency, especially at night when the yang is at its lowest, both in the body and in the environment. The Kidney yang deficiency influences the circulation of qi and blood to cause pain and coldness in the knee joints.

There is a feeling of being cold together with cold extremities, which indicates a general deficiency of yang. Cold is the main characteristic of the symptoms involving the Spleen and Kidney.

Fig. 5

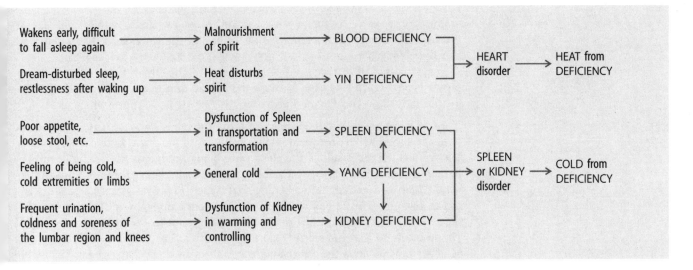

The patient has an inability to adapt to temperature changes because he suffers from both heat from deficiency and deficiency of yang. In cold weather the heat caused by the yin deficiency is too weak to keep the body warm and the patient's symptoms of cold become worse. When the weather is hot, the cold symptoms may improve slightly, but those related to heat will be intensified and the patient will not feel better. He is therefore averse to both heat and cold.

Patients with yang deficiency commonly have pale complexions, while those with yin deficiency often have a malar flush, especially in the afternoon. This patient's face is pale, but if he were observed throughout the day he might well develop a malar flush too.

The tongue body is red and the coating is dry and yellow, indicating the presence of heat. There is also yang deficiency, thus the tongue is dark rather than the typical fresh red associated with heat from deficiency.

The pulse on the right wrist reflects the health of the Lung, Spleen, and Kidney yang. On the left side the Heart, Liver, and Kidney yin can be assessed. Lung, Spleen, and Kidney yang control the yang and the qi, whereas the Heart, Liver, and Kidney yin control yin and blood. It is therefore possible to obtain information about the yang aspect from the right-hand pulse, and about the yin aspect from the left.

This patient has a slippery, forceless pulse on the right side indicating that the heat from deficiency is pushing the blood more rapidly than usual and causing a smooth, slippery flow. The pulse is forceless because there is also yang deficiency. The left side is sunken, slippery, and forceless showing yin and blood deficiency with the vessels being insufficiently filled. The third position on the right side is thin, reflecting the Kidney yang deficiency, while the very weak pulse felt on the first position of the left side indicates Heart yin deficiency.

Pattern of disease

There is no invasion by external pathogenic factors and the history is long, the main problem being insomnia; it is thus an interior pattern.

The patient has Heart yin deficiency leading to 'heat above', together with Spleen and Kidney yang deficiency resulting in 'cold below'; it is thus a pattern with both heat and cold.

There is deficiency of qi, blood, yin, and yang; it is thus a pattern of pure deficiency.

Additional notes

1. There may be some confusion regarding the cold pattern in this case, as the patient feels cold and has cold extremities, which might suggest an exterior pattern.

However, there is no history of invasion by pathogenic cold, and the patient has no aversion to cold. As such we must regard him as a person with a 'cold' constitution. The extremities are regarded as the end of the yang, such that when there is a deficiency the yang qi does not reach them and they become cold.

The location of heat or cold is determined by the Organ from which the symptoms originate. In this case, because the Spleen and Kidney are relatively lower in the body than the Heart, the pattern is one of heat above with cold below.

2. In case numbers 33 and 35 the symptom of dizziness was caused by deficiency of qi and blood with consequent malnourishment of the spirit. In this case, however, the dizziness is the result of the clear yang being unable to rise to the head. The patient not only complains of dizziness, but also of a heavy sensation around the head which is apparent on wakening, but which improves when he gets up and moves around. This is characteristic of dizziness caused by qi deficiency rather than blood deficiency. In health the clear yang rises to the head and the turbid yin descends so that the spirit is alert. This patient has Spleen qi deficiency, and as qi pertains to yang, the clear yang lacks sufficient support to rise up. The turbid yin remains in the head, resulting in a sensation of heaviness, which tends to improve when the patient moves about in the morning, as physical activity helps the yang qi circulate and rise.

3. Is urinary frequency only associated with a pattern of heat?

In the basic theory of this case (see above) the example of damp-heat in the Bladder was cited as a pattern of heat below. The symptoms were frequency and urgency with yellow urine and a scalding pain when urinating. Frequency is caused by the pathogenic heat draining out of the body in the urine. However, this patient has only frequency and nocturia, with no symptoms of heat. There is yang deficiency, so control of the Bladder is weakened, and less water than usual is reabsorbed because of the Kidney yang deficiency. The frequency in this case is thus part of a cold pattern.

4. The patient has a greasy tongue coating, thick in the middle and at the root. This indicates retention of damp-heat in the Spleen and Stomach, which is discussed in case number 34 (additional note no. 4).

Conclusion

1. According to the eight principles:
   Interior, heat above with cold below, deficient pattern.
2. According to Organ theory:
   Deficiency of Heart blood and yin.
   Deficiency of Spleen and Kidney yang.

Treatment principle

1. Nourish the Heart yin, remove the heat, and calm the spirit.
2. Tonify the Spleen and Kidney.

Selection of points

Sp-15 *(da heng)*
CV-6 *(qi hai)*
P-3 *(qu ze)*
an mian (N-HN-54)
H-9 *(shao chong)*
Sp-1 *(yin bai)*

Explanation of points

Sp-15 *(da heng)* tonifies the Spleen and regulates the qi. It also has the function of removing dampness caused by deficiency of Spleen qi or Spleen yang.

CV-6 *(qi hai)* tonifies the qi and Kidney and is one of the most important tonifying points. It also regulates the qi of the body, but this is secondary to its tonifying function.

P-3 *(qu ze)* removes the obstruction from the Heart channel, facilitating the circulation of qi. As the sea point on the Pericardium channel, it removes heat, especially from the blood level.

an mian (N-HN-54) is a good point for calming the spirit and pacifying the Heart. It helps dizziness, headache, and insomnia caused by disturbance of the spirit.

H-9 *(shao chong)* also calms the spirit.

Sp-1 *(yin bai)* regulates the Spleen and the blood.

Sp-1 *(yin bai)* and H-9 *(shao chong)*, both well points, are used together to calm the spirit and relieve dream-disturbed sleep caused by Heart and Spleen dysfunction.

Follow-up

At the time this patient was seen he had already received two months of acupuncture treatment without a favorable result. He was then treated 2-3 times a week for four weeks. His appetite and digestion gradually improved, and the coldness around his body diminished. His insomnia improved slightly. He received no treatment for two weeks due to pressure of work, and when he returned he had not regressed. He then received two more weeks' treatment with the same points, after which his complexion returned to normal, his dreaming diminished considerably, he had less nocturia, and his sleep pattern generally improved. His stools also became more formed. He was then treated for one week with both acupuncture and the following herbs:

Rhizoma Coptidis *(huang lian)*
Semen Zizyphi Spinosae *(suan zao ren)*
Radix Polygalae Tenuifoliae *(yuan zhi)*
Radix Angelicae Sinensis *(dang gui)*
Cortex Cinnamomi Cassiae *(rou gui)*
Rhizoma Atractylodis Macrocephalae *(bai zhu)*
Pericarpium Citri Reticulatae *(chen pi)*
Radix Astragali Membranacei *(huang qi)*
Sclerotium Poriae Cocos *(fu ling)*
Radix Codonopsitis Pilosulae *(dang shen)*
Radix Rehmanniae Glutinosae *(sheng di huang)*
Radix Dioscoreae Oppositae *(shan yao)*

After this he received only five treatments over two months. His energy was much improved and his tongue and pulse picture became more normal. The patient was very busy with his job and did not return for treatment after five months.

Diagnostic principles for insomnia

In clinical practice insomnia is a very common complaint. There are several different types of insomnia: there may be poor sleep, difficulty in falling asleep, dream-disturbed sleep, and premature awakening accompanied by difficulty in returning to sleep. In Chinese medicine the different manifestations of insomnia imply different pathological changes.

Physiology of sleep

In Chinese medicine sleeping and wakening reflect the cyclical change of yin and yang. When sleep occurs the yang becomes immersed in yin. At this time the yin governs the body. When the yang reemerges from yin, the person will wake up. At this time the yang governs the body. The cycle of yin and yang in the body corresponds to the yin and yang cycle in the environment. The yin and yang of the body is dynamic: as the environment changes so too will the yin and yang of the body. This relationship is manifested through the activity of the spirit: during the night the spirit gets into the yin and blood, and people become quiet and will fall asleep peacefully; during the day the spirit leaves the yin and blood, and people wake up and once again become active.

Disorders may occur if something influences the ability of the spirit to enter the yin. The disturbance may also occur if the spirit cannot peacefully remain in the yin and blood. These are two fundamental causes of insomnia.

Pathology of insomnia

There are four different types of sleep disorders in Chinese medicine:

1. Heat disturbing the spirit

The yang governs activity and movement of the spirit. Heat is a yang pathogenic factor, and will disturb the spirit to make it overactive and restless. There are two sources of this heat:

a) From the Organs which are close to the Heart. This will raise the Heart temperature and disturb the spirit.

b) The environment of the spirit can also be upset directly. This can occur when there is heat in the blood.

Fig. 6

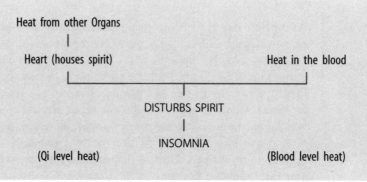

Heat may be caused by deficiency or an external pathogenic factor. The type of insomnia from heat will usually involve difficulty in falling asleep, restlessness, and sometimes a feverish sensation in the Heart. The disturbance of sleep by dreams and palpitations may also occur.

2. Malnourishment of the spirit

The activity of the spirit is supported by the nourishment from Heart blood. When the Heart blood is deficient, the spirit will lose nourishment and cause disorder in the Heart. The symptoms of this condition include early awakening accompanied by difficulty in returning to sleep. There may also be difficulty in falling asleep, but it is important to note that this will not be accompanied by restlessness, i.e., there is no heat.

3. Deficiency of spirit

Deficiency of spirit can also cause insomnia. According to the theory of yin and yang, the spirit is part of the yang-qi function, and the Heart blood is part of the yin aspect. The interdependence of yin and yang is indeed important. A disharmony of one will in theory lead to a dysfunction of the other. However in the clinical situation, sometimes only one aspect will malfunction. A good example is deficiency of spirit. This pattern will involve a lack of energy, palpitations, and a timid personality which is easily frightened.

The accompanying insomnia will result in poor sleep. Sometimes the patient may wake up several times a night. The disturbed sleep may be accompanied by nightmares or dreams of a frightening nature. This type of insomnia will not have any symptoms of blood deficiency, and can thus be distinguished from that type.

4. Other disorders

When insomnia is a secondary problem, differentiation must be cautious. For example, severe abdominal pain and painful obstruction can disturb one's sleep. When this occurs there is no need to look for any deeper cause of the insomnia—the pain is enough to keep one awake. For this type of insomnia the most important thing is to treat the underlying cause of the disorder. Only then will one's sleep improve.

Fig. 7

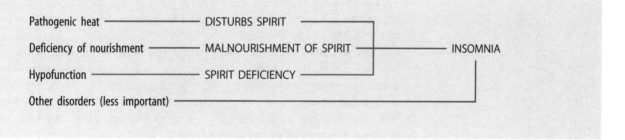

Classification of insomnia

In the clinical situation there are many different types of insomnia. A comprehensive list is provided in Fig. 8 below.

Key points in diagnosing insomnia

1. Heat disturbs the spirit

This type of insomnia is characterized by restlessness and palpitations. The restlessness makes it difficult to fall asleep. The harder the patient tries to sleep, the more restless he or she becomes. This can lead to a frustrating, vicious circle of increasing discomfort. The severe form of restlessness can be self-induced: when

Fig. 8

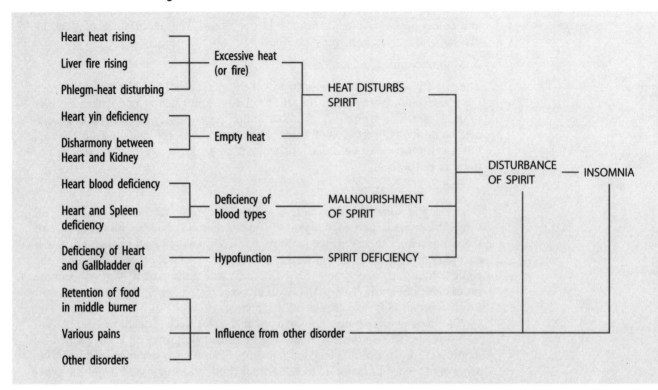

the patient tries unsuccessfully to sleep, they will often allow their emotions to make themselves even more restless. Some patients develop a conditioned form of restlessness: once it becomes time for sleep they will automatically become restless. In this case sleep can almost become a psychological burden. The patient will sometimes even be afraid to go to bed.

The disturbing heat can be excessive or deficient in nature. The excessive heat pattern will manifest in severe restlessness, irritability, dream-disturbed sleep, and even night-long insomnia. This type of patient will have many symptoms of an accompanying excessive heat pattern. The tongue will be red with a thick yellow coating. The pulse will tend to be forceful and rapid.

The heat from deficiency pattern will also manifest in restlessness, irritability, and dream-disturbed sleep, but the symptoms will be much less severe. The patient's general complaint may involve difficulty falling asleep, but the occurrence of night-long sleeplessness is very rare in this pattern. Accompanying symptoms will be hot in nature but quite mild, and in some patients heat may not even be too obvious. The tongue will be red and may be smaller and thinner. The tongue coating will be thin, yellow, and dry. The pulse will be thin and rapid.

2. Malnourishment of the spirit

This type of insomnia frequently exhibits a pattern of early awakening, after which the patient is unable to return to sleep. There will be no restlessness or irritability, hence there will be no palpable psychological discomfort, and the individual will awaken prematurely but remain peacefully lying in bed.

In the clinical situation there are two variations of this pattern. The patient may have Heart blood deficiency. In this type the insomnia will be accompanied by poor memory. In order to make this diagnosis the patient should exhibit blood deficiency symptoms, including pale face, pale tongue, pale finger nails, and a thin pulse.

There can also be a deficiency of the Heart and Spleen. This form of insomnia will be accompanied by general lassitude and daytime drowsiness. During the day the patient will complain of an unclear spirit. This may be accompanied by slight dizziness. The patient may also have a poor appetite, pale face, and pale tongue. The tongue coating will be white, and the pulse thin and forceless. These symptoms are caused by qi and blood deficiency.

3. Heart and Gallbladder qi deficiency

The main characteristic of this form of insomnia is poor quality of sleep. The sleep will be accompanied by nightmares. Once the nightmare is over the patient will usually fall asleep again quickly. This type of patient will commonly fall asleep easily and will not wake up prematurely. This problem is more common in people with timid personalities. They may develop anxiety and frighten easily. The insomnia may be accompanied by general manifestations of deficiency, e.g., a stifling sensation in the chest or shortness of breath. The tongue may be normal, but the pulse will be thin and forceless.

4. Other causes of insomnia

In this category the insomnia will be a secondary problem, and will consequently have no particular pattern of disease.

Fig. 9   The entire diagnostic procedure for insomnia is summarized in Fig. 9.

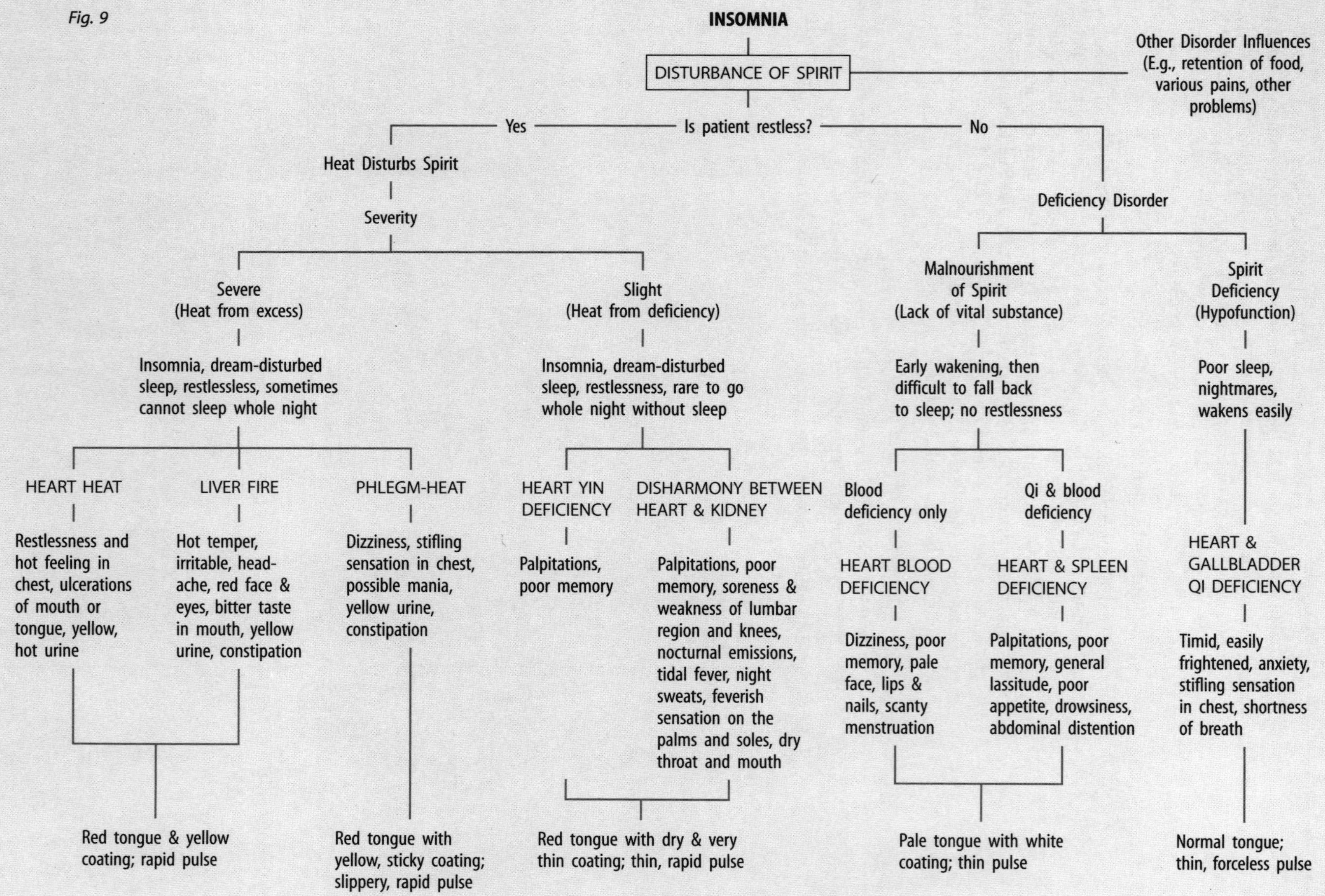

INSOMNIA

DISTURBANCE OF SPIRIT

Is patient restless?

Yes — **Heat Disturbs Spirit**

No — **Deficiency Disorder**

Other Disorder Influences (E.g., retention of food, various pains, other problems)

Heat Disturbs Spirit — Severity

Severe (Heat from excess)

Insomnia, dream-disturbed sleep, restlessless, sometimes cannot sleep whole night

- **HEART HEAT**
  Restlessness and hot feeling in chest, ulcerations of mouth or tongue, yellow, hot urine

- **LIVER FIRE**
  Hot temper, irritable, headache, red face & eyes, bitter taste in mouth, yellow urine, constipation

  Red tongue & yellow coating; rapid pulse

- **PHLEGM-HEAT**
  Dizziness, stifling sensation in chest, possible mania, yellow urine, constipation

  Red tongue with yellow, sticky coating; slippery, rapid pulse

Slight (Heat from deficiency)

Insomnia, dream-disturbed sleep, restlessness, rare to go whole night without sleep

- **HEART YIN DEFICIENCY**
  Palpitations, poor memory

- **DISHARMONY BETWEEN HEART & KIDNEY**
  Palpitations, poor memory, soreness & weakness of lumbar region and knees, nocturnal emissions, tidal fever, night sweats, feverish sensation on the palms and soles, dry throat and mouth

  Red tongue with dry & very thin coating; thin, rapid pulse

Deficiency Disorder

Malnourishment of Spirit (Lack of vital substance)

Early wakening, then difficult to fall back to sleep; no restlessness

- **Blood deficiency only**
  - **HEART BLOOD DEFICIENCY**
    Dizziness, poor memory, pale face, lips & nails, scanty menstruation

- **Qi & blood deficiency**
  - **HEART & SPLEEN DEFICIENCY**
    Palpitations, poor memory, general lassitude, poor appetite, drowsiness, abdominal distention

  Pale tongue with white coating; thin pulse

Spirit Deficiency (Hypofunction)

Poor sleep, nightmares, wakens easily

- **HEART & GALLBLADDER QI DEFICIENCY**
  Timid, easily frightened, anxiety, stifling sensation in chest, shortness of breath

  Normal tongue; thin, forceless pulse

Fig. 9

Palpitations

CASE 37: **Male, age 45**

Main complaint

Palpitations

History

The patient has complained of episodic palpitations with a rapid heart beat for over one year. Initially they occurred only rarely, but now they occur every few days, whenever he works too hard or does not take enough rest. During the onset, severe restlessness sets in, accompanied by shortness of breath and a stifling sensation in the chest. When he rests the symptoms gradually disappear.

Since the palpitations have developed his appetite has decreased and his sleep is poor. Bowel movements and urination are both normal. His complexion is dusky, lusterless, and pale.

Tongue

Slightly red body, thin, and white coating

Pulse

Forceless

Analysis of symptoms

1. Palpitations, poor sleep—disturbance of the spirit.
2. Stifling sensation in the chest, shortness of breath—deficiency of pectoral qi.
3. Poor appetite—Spleen qi deficiency.
4. Dark and pale complexion, forceless pulse—qi deficiency.

Basic theory of case

Palpitations represent the patient's subjective view that the heart is beating faster than usual, particularly when the heart rate is above the normal limit. This can occur episodically or continuously. Some patients feel anxious and restless and find it difficult to control themselves. There can also be episodic anxiety and restlessness, accompanied by a feverish sensation and sweating. Objectively the heart rate may or may not rise, but even when it doesn't it is still considered to be part of the palpitations category in traditional Chinese medicine.

The most common cause of palpitations is shock or fright. This type of palpitations usually disappears quickly, and then is of no clinical significance. If palpitations occur without a history of shock, it is always considered pathological.

Palpitations are one of the most common symptoms of a Heart disorder. Continuous palpitations are considered much more severe than episodic ones. Palpitations have many different causes, thus the diagnosis should only be made after analysis of all the symptoms.

Cause of disease

Qi deficiency

There are no external pathogenic factors involved in this case. The palpitations are closely related to overexertion, and when the patient rests the symptoms improve. He also has a stifling sensation in the chest, feels breathless, and has a forceless pulse. These symptoms indicate a level of qi deficiency which cannot support the normal function of the Heart.

Site of disease

Heart

Palpitations are the main evidence of a Heart disorder.

Pathological change

The Heart controls the blood, and the Heart qi has the function of circulating the blood in the vessels. When the Heart qi is abundant, the heart rate, rhythm, and force will be normal, allowing the blood to circulate and nourish the body.

This patient has Heart qi deficiency. The force of circulation has diminished, and the heart beat has become forceless and rapid in order to compensate for the deficiency of qi. This maintains the Heart's basic functions, but also causes the palpitations. The physical strain consumes the body's qi, and poor sleep leads to poor coordination of the body functions. These two factors combine to reduce the qi level and induce the palpitations. When the patient rests, the consumption of qi decreases, and this alleviates the patient's symptoms.

As discussed in the chapter on insomnia, the function of sleep is closely related to the Heart. This is because when the Heart qi is deficient, all the functions of the Heart are affected. This includes its function of housing the spirit. When this occurs it will manifest clinically as sleep disorders.

The qi of the chest is called pectoral qi (also known as ancestral qi, or *zōng qì*) and has two functions. It governs inhalation and exhalation, this being part of the function of the Lung qi. It also governs the circulation of blood, which is part of the Heart qi function. This patient suffers from Heart qi deficiency, which also produces a deficiency of pectoral qi. This leads to shortness of breath and a stifling sensation in the chest along with the palpitations.

Pectoral qi is formed from the yang of heaven which is inhaled by the Lung, and the qi of food essence which is produced by the Spleen. It therefore has a very close relationship with both Lung and Spleen qi. When the pectoral qi is weak it tries to compensate for this by 'pilfering' the qi of the Spleen. This forces the Spleen to work harder, which eventually injures the Spleen qi. Poor appetite is a clinical manifestation of this disorder. *See Fig. 1.*

The complexion is dusky, pale, and lusterless as a direct result of the Heart qi deficiency, because the Heart is unable to push the blood upwards to nourish the face. The forceless pulse is characteristic of qi deficiency.

Pattern of disease

There are no external pathogenic factors involved in this case. The site of disease is the Heart, so this is an interior pattern.

The patient has qi deficiency without any obvious imbalance of yin and yang. There are no symptoms to indicate the presence of either cold or heat.

There is no retention of pathogenic factors. The qi is deficient, and consequently this is a pattern of deficiency.

Additional notes

1. Does this patient have Lung or Spleen qi deficiency?

With pectoral qi deficiency there may be some effect upon the function of the Lung or Spleen. In this case the pectoral qi deficiency has been caused by Heart qi deficiency, and the patient complains of shortness of breath, a stifling sensation in the chest, and poor appetite. But the symptoms are mild and the influence is very slight. The symptoms relating to the Heart are much more significant, thus a diagnosis of Lung or Spleen qi deficiency would not be justified.

Fig. 1

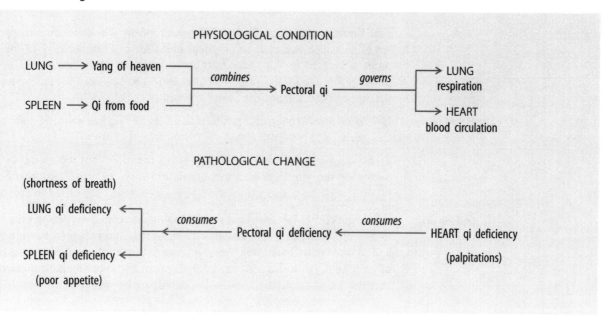

PHYSIOLOGICAL CONDITION

LUNG ——→ Yang of heaven ——┐
                            ├─ *combines* ——→ Pectoral qi —— *governs* ——→ LUNG respiration
SPLEEN ——→ Qi from food ——┘   └──→ HEART blood circulation

PATHOLOGICAL CHANGE

(shortness of breath)
LUNG qi deficiency ←──┐
                      ├── *consumes* ── Pectoral qi deficiency ←── *consumes* ── HEART qi deficiency
SPLEEN qi deficiency ←─┘   (palpitations)
(poor appetite)

2. What caused the Heart qi deficiency?

This may be due to several causes: a) congenital deficiency; b) injury to the qi caused by a chronic disorder; c) injury to the Heart as a result of some other Organ disorder; or d) sometimes the Heart qi can be injured by pathogenic factors.

This particular case involved a long history, and the onset was slow and gradual. This made it very difficult for the patient to remember the circumstances of onset, thus very little valuable information was obtained from the case history. We can say only that this patient has a primary Heart qi deficiency. He does not have any previous history of some other Organ disorder because the palpitations were the first symptom. The other symptoms, e.g., shortness of breath, occurred later. The most likely cause is either a congenital deficiency or injury to the qi as a result of a chronic disorder.

Conclusion

1. According to the eight principles:
   Interior, neither heat nor cold, deficiency pattern.

2. According to qi, blood, body fluids theory:
   Qi deficiency.

3. According to Organ theory:
   Heart qi deficiency.

Treatment principle

1. Reinforce the Heart qi.
2. Calm the spirit.

Selection of points

B-15 *(xin shu)*
B-13 *(fei shu)*
B-24 *(qi hai shu)*
H-7 *(shen men)*
Sp-6 *(san yin jiao)*

Explanation of points

Note that no front chest points were used in this case. This is because it is prudent to avoid points on the front of the trunk in patients with palpitations or anxiety. Puncturing these points can easily provoke panic attacks or extreme anxiety.

The combined use of B-15 *(xin shu)* and B-13 *(fei shu)* increases the qi of the

Heart and Lung. This promotes the pectoral qi of the upper burner. When the pectoral qi is sufficient the circulation of blood and qi will improve.

The Chinese name for B-24 *(qi hai shu)* means the back entrance point of the sea of qi, which makes it an excellent point for regulating the qi of the body. This point is located in the lower burner, whereas the other associated points in the prescription are in the upper burner. B-24 *(qi hai shu)* supports the actions of the upper points from the lower burner.

H-7 *(shen men)*, the source point of hand lesser yin, has a strong action in calming the spirit.

Sp-6 *(san yin jiao)* is the meeting point of the three foot yin channels. This point nourishes the yin, regulates the circulation of blood, and can also help prevent blood stasis. In conjunction with H-7 *(shen men)* it calms the spirit.

Follow-up

After one course of treatment consisting of six visits over two weeks, the palpitations were noticeably reduced and the insomnia and stifling sensation in the chest had disappeared. There was then a one-week break followed by two further courses of treatment, or twelve sessions in all. By then the appetite had returned to normal and the palpitations had virtually ceased, so he was able to return to work.

CASE 38: **Female, age 51**

Main complaint

Palpitations and toothache

History

The patient has a history of palpitations for several years. The toothache began last week.

Her general constitution is weak, as she has general lassitude, frequent bouts of episodic palpitations, and shortness of breath. Last week she developed painful, swollen gums. There is no bleeding from the gums, but the pain radiates to the neck. She has a dry mouth and throat and a desire to drink. Food intake is normal, but she has not defecated for three days, which is a new development. The patient has chronic sensations of cold and pain in the lower back and knee joints.

Tongue

Pale body, white, greasy tongue coating

Pulse

Wiry and slippery

Analysis of symptoms

1. Palpitations, shortness of breath—Heart qi deficiency.
2. Swollen and painful gums, dryness in the mouth, desire to drink, constipation—fire.
3. Feeling of cold and pain in the lower back and knee joints—cold.
4. Pale tongue—qi deficiency.
5. Slippery pulse—heat.

Basic theory of case

The antipathogenic factor *(zheng qi)* is the ability of the body to function normally, to ward off disease, and to recover from disorders or injuries when they occur. It is considered to be the harmonious interaction of many components of the body including the qi, blood, fluids, and essence, along with the various functions of the Organs, channels and collaterals. Protective qi is only a small part of the antipathogenic factor.

The term pathogenic factor covers a wide spectrum of disease-causing factors including 1) the six external factors (also known as pathogenic influences); 2) the seven emotional factors; 3) improper diet; 4) overwork and stress; 5) traumatic injury; and 6) Organ dysfunction which can lead to phlegm, pathogenic water, and/or blood stasis.

The onset of disease disturbs the normal physiological functions of the body, causing disharmony between yin and yang. This imbalance results in symptoms of disease. The occurrence and development of a disease is controlled by the relative strength of the pathogenic and antipathogenic factors. There is a group of symptoms which represents a deficiency of antipathogenic factor; together they constitute a pattern of deficiency. Another group of symptoms represents retention or invasion of pathogenic factors; together they constitute a pattern of excess. Not infrequently, patterns of excess and deficiency may occur in the same patient. This is referred to as a combination of excess and deficiency patterns.

Cause of disease

There are two causes in this case:

a) Pathogenic fire

The patient has red, swollen gums, dry mouth, and constipation indicating that the fire has risen up and blocked the channels, caused stagnation, and consumed the body fluids.

b) Deficiency of antipathogenic factor

There is shortness of breath, palpitations, general lassitude, and pain and cold in the lower back and knee joints. The tongue is pale. These symptoms indicate qi deficiency in the upper burner and yang deficiency in the lower burner.

Site of disease

Stomach, Heart, and Kidneys

The painful swollen gums and constipation indicate heat in the Stomach.
The palpitations and shortness of breath suggest a Heart disorder.
The pain and cold in the lower back and knee joints imply a Kidney disorder.

Pathological change

There are not many symptoms in this case, and they tend to be contradictory; it is therefore a complicated case. There is a combination of heat, cold, excess, and deficiency.

When approaching a case of this nature the symptoms must first be grouped into relevant categories before proceeding. Failure to do so increases the margin of error in diagnosis. In this case there are three groups of symptoms:

The first group is related to the weak constitution. The patient has lassitude, frequent palpitations, and shortness of breath. These are long-term symptoms resulting from Heart qi deficiency, and they represent a diminished level of energy in the blood, a common cause of palpitations. The pectoral qi of the chest is also weak, resulting in shortness of breath. The weak constitution and general lassitude are characteristic of qi deficiency.

The second group of symptoms includes chronic coldness and pain in the lower back and knee joints. These symptoms indicate internal cold caused by deficiency of Kidney yang. The lower back is known as the dwelling of the Kidney. The deficiency of Kidney yang signifies a loss in its warming function, which will affect the health of the lower back and knees and encourage the development of cold and pain. However, both of these symptoms are very slight, indicating that the degree of Kidney yang deficiency is not too severe.

The third group of symptoms includes the swollen and aching gums with pain that radiates to the neck, and the dry mouth with a desire to drink. There is also constipation. The symptoms are severe and are part of the patient's main complaint, although the history is very short. The yang brightness channel passes through the gums, and pain and swelling of the gums is usually associated with the yang brightness Organs. The Stomach yang brightness is rich in qi and blood; thus when there is fire in the Stomach, the pattern will be strong. The fire ascends upward along the channel, but the natural flow of the Stomach yang brightness channel is downward. The ascending fire collides with the descending qi and creates an obstruction in the channel. When this obstruction occurs in the gums it creates pain and swelling. The pain radiates downward along the channel.

The fire has also consumed the fluids, which explains the dry throat and thirst with a desire to drink. The injury to the body fluids in the Large Intestine causes constipation. The digestive function is hyperactive in the patient with Stomach fire. There is a Chinese proverb that is apropos: "A stove with a strong fire uses more fuel." Similarly, a patient with this disorder tends to eat more rather than less.

There are two groups of chronic symptoms in this case: Heart qi deficiency and Kidney yang deficiency. These two groups may appear to have little in common, but according to traditional pathology they may be closely connected. The Kidney yang is the root of the yang and qi of the whole body. When the Kidney yang is deficient it may affect the Heart, giving rise to symptoms of either Heart yang or Heart qi deficiency. This is one form of disharmony between fire (Heart) and water (Kidney). There is a possibility here that this may have occurred, although there is not enough evidence to support the theory. It is also possible that the two groups of symptoms are independent of one another.

It is impossible that the Kidney yang deficiency developed secondarily to the Heart qi deficiency. This is because a pattern of qi deficiency is not as severe as a pattern of yang deficiency. If the Kidney yang deficiency were to be caused by a Heart disorder, the pathology would be different. The Heart qi deficiency could degenerate into a Heart yang disorder, and if the problem persisted it would evolve into Kidney yang deficiency, as the yang of the upper burner can consume the yang of the lower burner.

The Stomach fire pattern is one of both heat and excess. The Kidney and Heart disorders are both deficient and cold. We can therefore discount the possibility of any disease relationship here.

Fig. 2

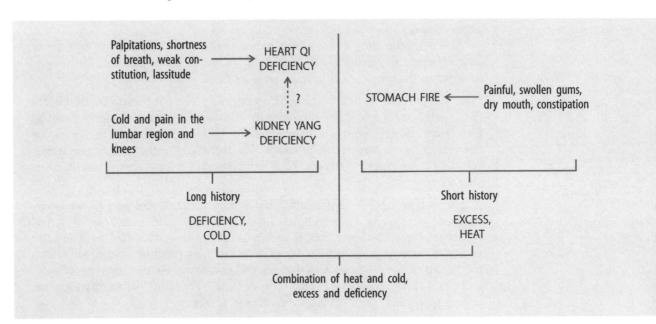

This case is a combination of heat and cold, excess and deficiency, and thus there are many possible manifestations on the tongue and pulse. The tongue here reflects a pattern of deficiency. The slippery pulse suggests a Stomach heat pattern because the heat increases the circulation of the blood. The wiry nature of the pulse indicates the presence of pain, which is caused by the pathogenic fire

The fire also retards the circulation of qi and blood and reduces the normal elasticity of the blood vessels. This is another reason why the pulse is wiry.

Pattern of disease

The site of disease is in the Organs, there is no invasion by pathogenic factors, and the patient thus has an interior pattern.

There is a combination of cold and heat. The coldness and pain in the lower back and knee joints represents Kidney yang deficiency, a form of cold. The dryness in the mouth, thirst, and constipation represent a pattern of heat.

There is also a combination of deficiency and excess. The deficiency pattern is comprised of the Heart qi and Kidney yang disorder. The swelling and pain of the gums reflects an excessive pattern.

Additional notes

1. Is the swelling and pain of the gums caused by fire from excess or deficiency?

Fire from excess in the Stomach is a common cause of swelling and pain of the gums. Fire from deficiency ('empty' fire) is a consequence of Kidney yin deficiency, as this causes a preponderance of yang, which can also cause the gums to swell. The symptoms and pathology of these two types of fire are different.

This patient has pain and swelling of the gums, indicating an excessive pattern. She displays no symptoms of Kidney yin deficiency, but does have symptoms of Kidney yang deficiency.

2. What is the cause of this patient's Stomach fire?

In the discussion on pathological change we already mentioned that the Stomach fire has no relationship to the other disorders. There are three common causes of this condition: a) over-consumption of hot and spicy food; b) invasion of the Stomach by internal or external heat; and c) stagnation of qi, leading to fire. This patient's history provides no insight into the cause of her condition, and therefore we cannot know.

3. What is the relevance of the greasy tongue coating?

A thick, greasy tongue coating indicates dampness, phlegm, and retention of food. Although this patient has such a tongue coating, as well as Kidney yang deficiency (which can give rise to dampness), because there are no other symptoms of dampness or phlegm the tongue coating is not of much significance.

Conclusion

1. According to the eight principles:
   Interior, mixed cold and heat, mixed excess and deficiency pattern.

2. According to etiology:
   Pathogenic fire.
   The deficiency developed from long-term illness.

3. According to channels and collaterals:
   Heat in the yang brightness channel.

4. According to Organ theory:
   Stomach fire rising up, Heart qi deficiency, and Kidney yang deficiency.

Treatment principle

1. Drain the Stomach fire.
2. Tonify the Heart qi.
3. The Kidney yang cannot be treated until the heat symptoms are resolved.

Selection of points

S-7 *(xia guan)*
S-44 *(nei ting)*
P-6 *(nei guan)*
CV-6 *(qi hai)*

Explanation of points

S-7 *(xia guan)* is an excellent choice for removing obstruction and heat from the channel. In this case it is also a local point for toothache.

S-44 *(nei ting)* is the spring point of the foot yang brightness channel. It clears Stomach fire and removes obstruction from the channel. It also drains heat from the two yang brightness Organs.

P-6 *(nei guan)* is a good point for regulating the Heart qi and disseminating the qi in the area of the chest. It also calms the spirit.

CV-6 *(qi hai)* is an excellent point for reinforcing the qi of the entire body and harmonizing the blood.

Combination of points

P-6 *(nei guan)* and CV-6 *(qi hai)* function to regulate the Heart and promote the qi of the entire body. By using the reinforcing method the Heart qi will improve. CV-6 *(qi hai)* supports this function from the lower burner.

Moxa is contraindicated at this time. Although applying moxa to CV-6 *(qi hai)* will promote the Kidney yang, it may also serve to aggravate the fire in the yang brightness Organs.

Follow-up

After the first visit the toothache subsided. The patient was treated daily for three days, after which the gums had returned to normal. The prescription was then changed to focus on the palpitations and the Kidney yang deficiency:

P-6 *(nei guan)*
CV-6 *(qi hai)* with moxa box
S-36 *(zu san li)* or K-3 *(tai xi)* in alternation

The patient was then treated three times a week. Each course consisted of ten treatments, followed by a three-day break. After two courses of treatment she had only occasional palpitations, and after five more treatments her energy was excellent and the palpitations had disappeared.

CASE 39: **Female, age 46**

Main complaint

Palpitations and shortness of breath

History

This woman has a history of chronic heart disease. The Western diagnosis was aortic insufficiency. She has a two-year history of frequent episodes of palpitations and shortness of breath. When she lies down the palpitations and shortness of breath are still severe. The heart rate exceeds 130 per minute. The patient cannot take any physical exercise, and the slightest exertion causes severe discomfort and loss of breath; even when seated she has great difficulty in breathing. She has been hospitalized many times with heart failure.

At present her breathing has become even worse with frequent wheezing when she attempts to move. She has both a cold appearance and cold limbs, and catches cold very easily. She complains of aching around the entire body. Her sleep is poor and she wakes easily during the night for no apparent reason. She has scanty, clear urine and constipation. Her bowel movements are only once every few days, but the stools are moist. Her complexion is dark and without luster.

Tongue

Pale, purplish body, white, greasy coating

Pulse

Thin and rapid

Analysis of symptoms

1. Severe, continuous palpitations, disturbed sleep—Heart deficiency.
2. Shortness of breath, difficulty breathing, wheezing with exertion— Lung qi deficiency.

3. Cold appearance and limbs, easily catches cold—yang deficiency.

4. General aching—poor circulation of qi and blood.

5. Dark, lusterless face, pale, purplish tongue—blood stasis.

6. White, greasy tongue coating—damp-cold.

7. Thin pulse—deficiency.

Basic theory of case

The yang deficiency pattern is a very common one in the clinic. The yang warms the body and controls the temperature. Thus when this function is impaired symptoms of cold will appear, such as a cold appearance, feeling of being cold, and cold extremities or limbs.

The Kidney yang is the root of the body's yang and thus has a strong influence over all the Organs and body tissues. Typical symptoms of Kidney yang deficiency are said to stem from failure of the fire at the gate of vitality *(mìng mén huǒ)*. Spleen and Heart yang deficiency patterns also display cold symptoms, but each exhibits a distinct pattern of disease.

There are several keys to distinguishing among the various types of yang deficiency. In addition to the obvious symptoms of cold, the patient with severe palpitations is suffering from a pattern of Heart yang deficiency. The patient with anorexia, abdominal distention or pain, and watery stools has Spleen yang deficiency. If there is cold in the lower back and knee joints, it is a pattern of Kidney yang deficiency.

Fig. 3

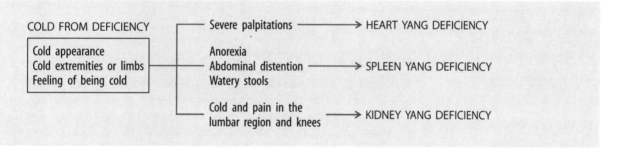

Cause of disease

1. Deficiency of yang.
2. Blood stasis.

The patient has cold limbs and a feeling of being cold, both of which are obvious symptoms of yang deficiency. The body consequently loses its ability to adequately warm itself.

The face is dark and lusterless. There is general aching around the body and a pale, purplish tongue. These signs suggest poor circulation of blood which has led to blood stasis.

Site of disease

Heart and Lungs

The severe palpitations and disturbed sleep represent involvement of the Heart.

The wheezing and difficulty in breathing suggest involvement of the Lungs.

Pathological change

The Heart qi and the Heart yang are both yang in nature. They share similar physical functions, like circulating the blood, but the Heart yang also has a warming function. It warms the spirit, vessels, and body through efficient blood circulation. The Heart qi does not have this function. The early stage of a Heart disorder involves qi deficiency, but if prolonged the pattern will transform into Heart yang deficiency. The principal manifestation involves a further deterioration of the original symptoms, with the addition of symptoms associated with internal cold.

In the early stages this patient had only Heart qi deficiency, but gradually the condition of the Heart worsened, leading to the emergence of Heart yang deficiency. As this continued the blood circulation became worse. This explains why the palpitations became more severe. Rest will usually relieve the consumption of Heart qi, but not Heart yang deficiency. This explains why rest in this case has not reduced the severity of the palpitations.

The Heart yang deficiency creates internal cold, impairing the warmth and nourishment provided to the spirit. This results in a particular type of poor sleep that is common in very sick patients. The patient may wake feeling scared, without having had a nightmare. The pathological change in this pattern is different from the insomnia caused by Heart blood or yin deficiency.

Heart yang deficiency can also upset the circulation of blood in the body: the level of qi in the blood is diminished, and the internal cold constricts the vessels. The combination of these two factors can cause blood stasis; the patient's dark, lusterless complexion and pale, purplish tongue are manifestations of this phenomenon. Her general aching is due to an insufficiency of qi in the channels and poor blood circulation. The cold appearance and cold limbs are the result of interior cold.

Fig. 4

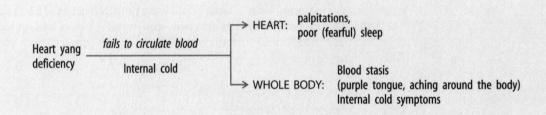

The Heart and Lungs are both located in the chest, and the foundation of their health is based on the strength of the pectoral qi. The chronic nature of this patient's illness has severely injured the Heart qi, and in order to compensate for this deficiency, the pectoral qi is consumed by the Heart. The Lung qi also continues to decline, causing wheezing and great difficulty in breathing.

The deficiency of Lung qi impairs the dissemination of protective qi, and the body's resistance to disease is weakened accordingly, making it easy for the patient to catch cold.

The white, greasy tongue coating and the thin pulse suggest a pattern of interior cold and deficiency.

Pattern of disease

The site of disease is in the Heart and Lungs, and this is accordingly an interior pattern.

This patient has developed internal cold from yang deficiency. The cold limbs and other signs of cold indicate a pattern of cold.

The palpitations, shortness of breath, and wheezing on exertion indicate a pattern of deficiency.

Additional notes

1. Does this patient at present have an exterior pattern?

The patient does have a very poor level of Lung qi, and her ability to resist the invasion of pathogenic factors is greatly reduced. This explains why she has frequent colds, an exterior pattern of disease.

However, according to her case history there was no exposure to cold. Her cold appearance and limbs are consistent with a pattern of internal cold, and there is no aversion to cold. Thus there is no exterior pattern at this time.

2. Is there a pattern of heat in this case?

The diagnosis was a pattern of cold, yet she has a rapid pulse, which is normally associated with a heat pattern. In this case, however, the rapid pulse is closely associated with the Heart yang deficiency. Because the Heart yang is nearly exhausted, it tries to compensates by pumping out more blood. The heart rate is over 130 beats per minute, but the force of the pulse is very weak. Thus, although the pulse is rapid, there is no heat pattern in evidence. (The rapid heart rate does not help the circulation of blood. The poor circulation of blood and internal cold leads to symptoms of blood stasis.)

3. Why is there an abnormal pattern of urination and constipation?

Internal cold caused by yang deficiency may allow pathogenic water or dampness to be retained in the body. This type of patient therefore frequently has clear, abundant urine and loose or watery stools. Here by contrast the patient has the opposite condition in which the urine output is reduced and bowel movements occur only once every few days. This is a severe form of yang deficiency which is not commonly seen in the clinic.

The yang qi warms and transforms water into fluids. When the yang qi is deficient this function may decline or cease altogether. Urination and defecation are the two principal means by which excessive water is discharged from the body, yet these two functions are likewise supported and controlled by the yang qi. Severe yang deficiency allows internal cold to become very strong, and the activity of qi is then profoundly affected. The dampness or pathogenic water becomes congealed or 'frozen' by the intense cold. This leads to a reduction in the amount of urine and the frequency of bowel movements. However, the urine is still clear in color and the stools are moist. If this patient had a heat pattern the stools would be dry and less frequent, while the urine would be yellow and reduced in quantity.

4. Is there a pattern of excess in this case?

Blood stasis is an excessive pathogenic factor. In the section on pathological change the poor circulation and blood stasis were discussed, so one might reasonably ask whether there is a combination of excess and deficiency. However, because the manifestations of blood stasis are not very strong, we attach less significance to this factor.

Conclusion	1. According to the eight principles: Interior, cold, deficient pattern. 2. According to Organ theory: Deficiency of Heart yang. Deficiency of Lung qi.
Treatment principle	1. Warm and tonify the Heart yang. 2. Tonify the Lung qi.
Selection of points	P-6 *(nei guan)* on one side L-9 *(tai yuan)* on one side CV-12 *(zhong wan)* CV-6 *(qi hai)* with warm needle S-36 *(zu san li)* with warm needle
Explanation of points	P-6 *(nei guan)* is a good choice for regulating the qi of the chest and Stomach and opening up the chest by removing the obstruction from this area. This point is considered to be a very important one for relieving chest pain and palpitations. It is the connecting point of the hand terminal yin channel, and allows access to the qi of the Triple Burner channel. P-6 *(nei guan)* also has a strong effect in calming the spirit. L-9 *(tai yuan)* is the source point of the hand greater yin channel. This point tonifies and regulates the Lung qi and helps promote the circulation of blood, as it is also the influential point for the blood vessels.

CV-12 *(zhong wan)*, CV-6 *(qi hai)*, and S-36 *(zu san li)* are all very important points for the tonification of qi and yang. When a patient is very weak, points from the middle and lower burner may be used to support the upper burner. Moreover, these three points reinforce the qi of the entire body, not just of the individual Organs.

This patient is very weak and the yang qi is seriously depleted. When treating this type of patient the less needles used, the better; there will be less discomfort and the antipathogenic factor will not be placed at risk. The associated points would commonly be used for this type of patient. However, they cannot be used here because this woman cannot lie on her back, stomach, or side. The only reasonable position is semi-supine with pillows propping her up, thus this group of points was chosen.

Follow-up

The patient was treated 2-3 times a week for four weeks. At the end of this time her heart rate had been lowered to about 100 per minute, and her dyspnea had improved. She continued treatment twice weekly for an additional three months. Her urine increased in quantity, her complexion became less pale, and the palpitations were less evident, although her heart rate remained rather rapid. She was able to do a reasonable amount of work in the house.

About six months later she caught cold and was hospitalized with severe heart failure. She had no further acupuncture treatments.

CASE 40: **Female, age 63**

Main complaint

Palpitations with anxiety

History

This patient has had recurrent anxiety attacks accompanied by palpitations for the past two years. Besides palpitations the patient has also experienced episodes of irritability, a stifling sensation in the chest, and shortness of breath.

Ten days ago after an emotional upset the symptoms recurred, but this time they were worse than usual. The patient complains of an episodic feverish sensation rising upwards to the head, and accompanied by sweating. She is not thirsty and prefers cold food, but her appetite is poor. There is no abdominal discomfort. The restlessness makes it difficult for her to fall asleep. She complains of coldness and pain in the lower back. Urination and bowel movements are normal.

Tongue

Slight red body, thin and white coating

Pulse

Thin

Analysis of symptoms

1. Palpitations, restlessness, insomnia, irritability—Heart yin deficiency.
2. Stifling sensation in the chest, shortness of breath—pectoral qi deficiency.
3. Feverish sensation with sweating—rising of heat from deficiency.
4. Poor appetite with a preference for cold food—Spleen deficiency.
5. Coldness and pain in the lower back—cold.
6. Thin pulse—deficiency.

Basic theory of case

Emotional factors play an important role in the onset and development of disease, especially when the emotion is continuous. In most cases emotional pathogenic factors attack the Heart and the Liver, but sometimes the Lung, Spleen, and Kidney are also affected.

The Heart is said to house the spirit and govern all vital psychological activities. The Heart therefore has a strong influence over perception, cognition, and consciousness. When the Heart function is disturbed, a wide variety of psychological symptoms may appear. Conversely, intense emotional upsets can disturb the function of the Heart.

The Liver governs the free flow of qi. The circulation and activity of qi around the entire body is maintained by the Liver. If this function is impaired, the patient will often develop irritability and depression. Conversely, severe and sudden emotional change can disturb the function of the Liver.

When there is excessive worry or pensiveness, the Spleen qi can stagnate or decline. Grief is the emotion associated with the Lung, thus excessive grieving will consume the Lung qi. The onset of extreme fear attacks the Kidneys, disrupting the function of Kidney qi.

Clinically speaking, an emotional factor does not always affect its corresponding Organ. For example, on a theoretical level thinking too much should injure the Spleen; in practice, however, it may injure both the Spleen and the Heart, or the Spleen, Heart, and Liver. The correct diagnosis can therefore only be made on the basis of the individual's own symptom pattern.

Cause of disease	**Emotional pathogenic factor** This patient has a history of palpitations and an anxious sensation in the chest. Before the latest episode the patient had an obvious flare of emotion in which she became angry, and afterwards suffered from depression. This is a strong indication that the problem was caused by an emotional pathogenic factor.
Site of disease	**Heart** The insomnia, palpitations, and feeling of restlessness in the chest are the main evidence suggesting Heart involvement.
Pathological change	Palpitations can be caused by several different factors, including Heart yin and Heart blood deficiency, or Heart yang and Heart qi deficiency. In this case there is a long history of irritability and anxiety, which is accompanied by palpitations. This group of symptoms suggests Heart yin deficiency, which generated heat from deficiency in the body, disturbing the spirit and causing restlessness and irritability. The insomnia pattern in this case involves restlessness and difficulty in falling asleep, symptoms which are characteristic of heat disturbing the spirit. The heat from deficiency ascends, and the patient complains of a hot sensation or flushes rising episodically to the head. The heat pushes the fluids outward in the form of sweat. In general, the typical manifestations of ascending heat from deficiency include 1) heat rising rapidly upwards from the body to the head; 2) a red complexion; 3) sweating on the forehead or entire body; and 4) severe restlessness. Usually, after a certain period of time, these symptoms will naturally decline, but will then recur from time to time. This is called heat from deficiency blazing upwards *(xū huǒ shàng yán)*. The chronic nature of the patient's Heart disorder consumes the pectoral qi of the chest, causing the stifling sensation in the chest and the shortness of breath. The Spleen is the primary source of blood and qi. The Heart yin and Heart blood are dependent upon the food essence from the Spleen, thus when the Heart yin is deficient it tends to consume greater quantities of the Spleen's food essence. If this situation persists the Spleen will eventually become deficient. This patient only has a poor appetite without abdominal discomfort, and the bowel movements, urination, and tongue are all normal. This indicates a mild degree of Spleen deficiency. If the patient is not treated, a pattern of full Spleen deficiency will eventually emerge.
Pattern of disease	In this case the onset was caused by emotional upset, and the site of disease is in the Heart. It is thus an interior pattern.

The patient is anxious, irritable, prefers cold food, experiences hot flushes, and sweats. This suggests a heat pattern.

The patient has a two-year history of palpitations, the pulse is thin, and there are no symptoms suggesting invasion of a pathogenic factor. It is therefore a pattern of deficiency.

Additional notes

1. How do we diagnose the true cause of the palpitations in a case of deficiency?

As previously mentioned, palpitations are a symptom common to all four Heart deficiency disorders. The deficiency of Heart qi and yang leads to palpitations, which are a direct result of the lack of energy. Accompanying symptoms will include a stifling sensation in the chest, shortness of breath, and general lassitude.

The palpitations caused by Heart blood deficiency or Heart yin deficiency will be accompanied by symptoms of insufficient nourishment of the spirit, or heat disturbing the spirit. These include poor memory, anxiety, dream-disturbed sleep, and insomnia.

This patient has anxiety, and her spirit is disturbed by heat from deficiency. She also suffers from shortness of breath and a stifling sensation in the chest. We cannot eliminate the possibility that the chronic yin deficiency has given rise to Heart qi deficiency, but at the moment the qi deficiency disorder is very mild and *Fig. 5* is not the main problem.

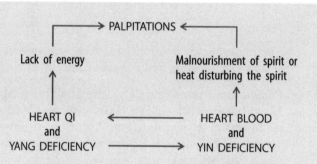

2. What type of Spleen deficiency is evident in this case?

The major Spleen symptoms are a poor appetite and a preference for cold food. These two symptoms could indicate deficiency of Spleen yin, but there are not enough other symptoms to support such a finding. Moreover, the tongue shows no signs of Spleen yin deficiency. As we mentioned earlier, the Spleen disorder is very mild. As yet no independent Spleen pattern has materialized. We therefore simply call this Spleen deficiency since we cannot pinpoint which aspect of the Spleen is deficient.

3. Is there Kidney yang deficiency in this case?

The coldness in the lower back has two possible origins: Kidney yang deficiency or retention of cold in the channel. A Kidney yang disorder will be accompanied by lumbar weakness and soreness, and this feeling may also be experienced on the lower limbs. The retention of pathogenic cold is a pattern of excess in which the patient will not have weakness in the affected area.

This patient has no weakness in the lower back, thus her condition is one of excess. However, because these symptoms are not closely related to the patient's main complaint, no further examination of these symptoms was made in this case.

Conclusion

1. According to the eight principles:
   Interior, heat, deficient pattern.

2. According to etiology:
   Emotional pathogenic factor.

3. According to Organ theory:
   Heart yin deficiency.

Treatment principle

1. Nourish the Heart yin.
2. Clear the heat.
3. Calm the spirit.

Selection of points

hua tuo jia ji (M-BW-35) at T4, T5, T9, T11, and T12
P-6 *(nei guan)* on one side
TB-5 *(wai guan)* on one side
Sp-4 *(gong sun)* on both sides

Explanation of points

Hua tuo jia ji (M-BW-35): The function of these points is similar to that of the associated points, but they are safer to puncture and easier to manipulate. This greater freedom in needle manipulation tends to enhance the therapeutic result. They have proven to be very useful for calming the spirit, and are often used when there is anxiety, worry, insomnia, and subjective feelings of abnormality.

There are many ways to select these points. One method is according to the corresponding associated points, and this is the method we used in this case. (An explanation of the other methods is beyond the scope of this case study.) We used the points on the same level as B-14, B-15, B-18, B-20, and B-21 which affect the Pericardium, Heart, Liver, Spleen, and Stomach respectively. This group of points promotes the function of the Heart and the middle burner, and calms the spirit and the patient's restlessness.

P-6 *(nei guan)* and TB-5 *(wai guan)* are both connecting points. P-6 *(nei guan)* calms the spirit and regulates the qi of the middle-upper burner. TB-5 *(wai guan)*, manipulated with a reducing method, helps to draw heat from the Pericardium channel. In this particular case, P-6 *(nei guan)* was needled on the left and TB-5 *(wai guan)* on the right.

In Chinese medicine, the left side is associated with yang and the right with yin in males. In females, it is just the opposite. This case refers to a female patient, thus TB-5 *(wai guan)* as a yang channel point is used on the right side, and P-6 *(nei guan)* as a yin channel point is used on the left.

Sp-4 *(gong sun)* is another connecting point which regulates the qi of the middle burner.

Combination of points

P-6 *(nei guan)* and Sp-4 *(gong sun)* are used together to relieve disorders of the middle and upper burners. The patient has severe restlessness in this case, and if the qi is regulated effectively, the heat will be eliminated.

Follow-up

This patient was treated three times weekly, one course consisting of six treatments with a five day break between courses. After the first course the anxiety was gone and she was sleeping well, but she still experienced coldness and pain in the lower back. After three more visits almost all her symptoms subsided, but for the next six months she occasionally experienced feelings of anxiety or palpitations which settled down after one or two treatments.

Diagnostic principles for deficiency patterns involving the five yin organs

Deficiency patterns imply an insufficiency of antipathogenic factors including yin, yang, qi, blood, vital essence, and body fluids. The cause may either be congenital (also known as pre-heaven) or acquired (post-heaven). Acquired deficiency can result from improper diet, stress (either mental or physical), trauma, or disease.

Clinically speaking, patterns of deficiency can occur in combination with patterns of excess, but for the purposes of this discussion we are concentrating primarily on instances of pure deficiency. When a deficient pattern is present there is invariably a long history, the disease has reached a late or chronic stage, and it has penetrated to the interior. The primary pathological change is malnourishment of the Organs.

1. Basic types of deficiency patterns

According to yin-yang theory, qi and yang relate to function and are associated with yang, whereas yin and blood are substantive and are associated with yin. Deficiencies of qi, yang, blood, and yin are the most common patterns seen in the clinic. These four patterns form the basis of understanding deficiencies in the yin Organs. Associated symptoms and key points for diagnosis are summarized below.

QI DEFICIENCY AND YANG DEFICIENCY

QI DEFICIENCY PATTERN	YANG DEFICIENCY PATTERN
General lassitude or fatigue, spontaneous sweating, weak voice, shortness of breath, symptoms worsen with physical movement or work, pale tongue, white coating, forceless pulse	General lassitude or fatigue, weak voice, shortness of breath, feeling of being cold, cold extremities, pale and flabby tongue with tooth marks, sunken, slow, and forceless pulse

Key points for diagnosis

These patterns both involve fatigue or general lassitude, shortness of breath, reluctance to speak, and a forceless pulse. The whole body is lacking in energy and the Organs are in a state of hypofunction.

In the case of yang deficiency the patient also looks cold, complains of feeling cold, and has cold extremities. The tongue is soft and flabby, and the pulse is slow. The body does not produce enough heat. These symptoms are absent from the pattern of qi deficiency. Qi deficiency symptoms plus the cold symptoms will therefore form the pattern of yang deficiency. In practice, qi deficiency may evolve into yang deficiency.

BLOOD DEFICIENCY AND YIN DEFICIENCY

BLOOD DEFICIENCY PATTERN	YIN DEFICIENCY PATTERN
Dizziness, insomnia, numbness on the hands and feet, pale face, nails, lips, and tongue, white coating, thready pulse. In women a long menstrual cycle, scanty and pink bloody discharge, or amenorrhea.	Dizziness, insomnia, malar flush, night sweats, tinnitus, feverish sensation in the palms and soles, anxiety, dry mouth and throat, red tongue with very thin coating, thready and rapid pulse

Key points for diagnosis

These patterns both involve dizziness, insomnia, and a thin pulse, indicating that the Organs and tissues are malnourished and that their physiological function is disturbed. Patients with blood deficiency will also have a pale complexion, pallor of the nails and lips, and a pale tongue, indicating that the blood is inadequate to nourish the whole body.

A patient with yin deficiency will experience malar flush, night sweats, restlessness, and afternoon fevers, as there is an imbalance between yin and yang, and hence a preponderance of yang or heat from deficiency (also known as 'empty' heat).

It should be noted that, unlike the relationship between qi and yang deficiency, yin deficiency does *not* represent a further development of blood deficiency, and one does not progress to the other.

The entire diagnostic procedure for these four patterns is set forth in the following chart.

Fig. 6

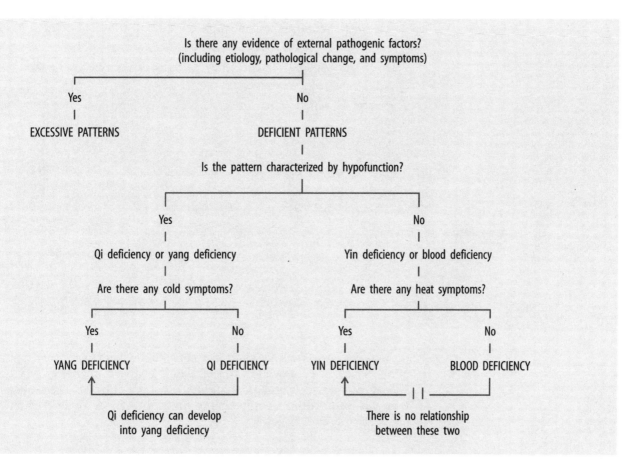

2. Basic symptoms involving deficiency of the five yin Organs

The five yin Organs have different functions. Thus, when an imbalance arises, each exhibits a different group of symptoms.

HEART

The Heart controls the vessels and houses the spirit. Symptoms of imbalance include palpitations, anxiety, insomnia, and poor memory.

LUNG

The Lung controls the qi of the entire body and governs respiration. When its function of dispersing and descending is impaired the patient will mainly show symptoms involving cough and asthma.

SPLEEN

The Spleen is responsible for the transformation and transportation of food and water metabolism. It also controls the muscles and the limbs. Symptoms of imbalance mainly affect the digestive system, e.g., poor appetite, abdominal distention, and loose stools. In addition the muscles may lose their nourishment and the patient will complain of general lassitude and fatigue and weakness of the limbs.

LIVER | The Liver stores the blood, controls the sinews, and opens through the eyes. The Liver channel passes through the hypochondriac region, and there may thus be discomfort or distention in the hypochondriac region or the intercostal spaces. There may also be visual disturbances, such as blurring of vision, and the nails may become thin, dry, and brittle. Numbness of the trunk or limbs may occur.

KIDNEY | The Kidney stores the vital essence and governs reproduction. It controls the bones and also urination and defecation. Kidney deficiency is reflected in such symptoms as soreness and weakness of the lower back and knee joints, urinary disorders, sexual dysfunction, or problems with defecation.

This list should make it possible to identify which yin Organ is suffering deficiency.

3. Diagnostic method for deficiency patterns of the five yin Organs

a) Determine which yin Organ is affected.
b) Determine which pattern of deficiency is present.

	QI DEFICIENCY	YANG DEFICIENCY	BLOOD DEFICIENCY	YIN DEFICIENCY
HEART	Heart qi deficiency	Heart yang deficiency	Heart blood deficiency	Heart yin deficiency
LUNG	Lung qi deficiency	--------	--------	Lung yin deficiency
SPLEEN	Spleen qi deficiency	Spleen yang deficiency	--------	Spleen yin deficiency
LIVER	--------	--------	Liver blood deficiency	Liver yin deficiency
KIDNEY	Kidney qi deficiency	Kidney yang deficiency	Kidney essence deficiency	Kidney yin deficiency

It should be noted from the chart that not all of the yin Organs have four patterns of deficiency. The Lung and Liver have only two, and the Spleen has three. The Kidney may have deficiency of vital essence, but not of blood. The missing patterns were not recorded historically, and in practice rarely occur in the clinic except under bizarre circumstances.

1. HEART DEFICIENCY PATTERNS

PATTERN	COMMON SYMPTOMS	DISTINGUISHING SYMPTOMS
HEART QI DEFICIENCY	↑ Palpitations, anxiety, pale tongue, forceless pulse	General lassitude or fatigue, suffocating sensation in the chest, shortness of breath, spontaneous sweating, symptoms worsen with physical movement, pale tongue, white coating, forceless pulse
HEART YANG DEFICIENCY	↓	Symptoms of qi deficiency and feeling of being cold, cold extremities, pale and flabby tongue, white and moist coating, sunken, slow, and forceless pulse
HEART BLOOD DEFICIENCY	↑ Palpitations, anxiety, insomnia, dream-disturbed sleep, thin pulse	Pale and lusterless face, pale lips and tongue, white tongue coating, forceless pulse
HEART YIN DEFICIENCY	↓	Afternoon fever or feverish sensation in palms and soles or dry mouth and throat, red tongue with thin coating, thin and rapid pulse

2. LUNG DEFICIENCY PATTERNS

PATTERN	COMMON SYMPTOMS	DISTINGUISHING SYMPTOMS
LUNG QI DEFICIENCY	Weak cough or asthma, white and clear phlegm	General lassitude, shortness of breath, weak voice, spontaneous sweating, the symptoms worsen with physical movement, pale tongue and white coating, forceless pulse
LUNG YIN DEFICIENCY	Cough with scanty phlegm or without phlegm, or scanty blood-stained phlegm	Afternoon fevers, night sweats, feverish sensation in the chest, palms, and soles, dry mouth and throat, red tongue with very little coating, thin and rapid pulse

3. SPLEEN DEFICIENCY PATTERNS

PATTERN	COMMON SYMPTOMS	DISTINGUISHING SYMPTOMS
SPLEEN QI DEFICIENCY	Poor appetite, abdominal distention worsens after taking food, loose stools, pale tongue, forceless pulse	General lassitude or fatigue, shortness of breath, weak voice, symptoms worsen with physical movement, pale tongue, white coating, forceless pulse
SPLEEN YANG DEFICIENCY		Qi deficiency symptoms and feeling of being cold, cold extremities or limbs, coldness and pain in the abdomen, pale and flabby tongue, white and moist coating, sunken, slow, and forceless pulse
SPLEEN YIN DEFICIENCY	Hungry but appetite is poor, dull abdominal pain	Dry mouth and throat, dry stool, red tongue, very thin coating or partly peeled coating, thin and rapid pulse

4. LIVER DEFICIENCY PATTERNS

PATTERN	COMMON SYMPTOMS	DISTINGUISHING SYMPTOMS
LIVER BLOOD DEFICIENCY	Discomfort in the inter-costal and hypochondriac regions, blurred vision, dizziness, tinnitus, wiry and thin pulse	Pale and lusterless face, dry and brittle nails, numbness on the hands and feet, pale lips and tongue, white coating, wiry and thin pulse
LIVER YIN DEFICIENCY		Afternoon fevers, night sweats, feverish sensation in the palms and soles, anxiety, dryness in the mouth and throat, red tongue with little coating, wiry, thin, rapid pulse

5. KIDNEY DEFICIENCY PATTERNS

PATTERN	COMMON SYMPTOMS	DISTINGUISHING SYMPTOMS
KIDNEY QI DEFICIENCY		General lassitude or fatigue, frequent urine or enuresis or incontinence of urine, involuntary emissions in men, excessive, clear, and lucid leukorrhea in women, pale tongue, white coating, forceless pulse
KIDNEY YANG DEFICIENCY	Soreness and weakness of the lumbar region and knee joints, urinary symptoms, or reproduc-tive disorder	General lassitude or fatigue, feeling of being cold, cold extremities or limbs, clear urine with increased quantity, loose or watery stools, edema, impotence in men, coldness in the lower abdomen and infertility in women, pale and flabby tongue, white and moist coating, sunken, slow, and forceless pulse
KIDNEY ESSENCE DEFICIENCY		Retarded development, early degeneration, sexual disability, slim tongue, thin pulse
KIDNEY YIN DEFICIENCY		Afternoon fevers, night sweats, feverish sensation in the palms and soles, anxiety, malar flush, dry mouth and throat, involuntary emissions with dream-disturbed sleep in men, scanty menstruation or amenorrhea in women, red tongue, very thin coating, thin and rapid pulse

Fig. 7

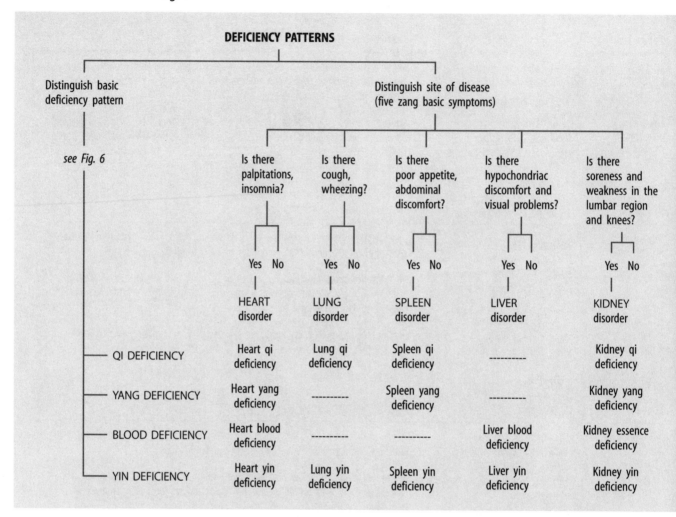

	HEART disorder	LUNG disorder	SPLEEN disorder	LIVER disorder	KIDNEY disorder
QI DEFICIENCY	Heart qi deficiency	Lung qi deficiency	Spleen qi deficiency	---------	Kidney qi deficiency
YANG DEFICIENCY	Heart yang deficiency	---------	Spleen yang deficiency	---------	Kidney yang deficiency
BLOOD DEFICIENCY	Heart blood deficiency	---------	---------	Liver blood deficiency	Kidney essence deficiency
YIN DEFICIENCY	Heart yin deficiency	Lung yin deficiency	Spleen yin deficiency	Liver yin deficiency	Kidney yin deficiency

Notes | Palpitations mainly occur in Heart deficiency patterns, but can also be seen in some excessive patterns, such as Heart blood stasis. Clinically, of course, there may be deficiency of two or more yin Organs together, and deficiency may occur with excess.

Select Bibliography

Anonymous. *Yellow Emperor's Inner Classic: Basic Questions (Huang di nei jing su wen)* 黄帝内经素问. Beijing: People's Health Publishing Company, 1956. [Originally written around 1st century B.C.]

Anonymous. *Yellow Emperor's Inner Classic: Vital Axis (Huang di nei jing ling shu)* 黄帝内经灵枢. Beijing: People's Health Publishing Company, 1956. [Originally written around 1st century B.C.]

Deng Tie-Tao. *Traditional Chinese Medical Diagnostics (Zhong yi zhen duan xue)* 中医诊断学. Shanghai: Shanghai Science & Technology Press, 1984.

Huang-Fu Mi. *Systematic Classic of Acupuncture and Moxibustion (Zhen jiu jia yi jing)* 针灸甲乙经. Beijing: People's Health Publishing Company, 1956. [Originally written in 3rd century A.D.]

Li Ding. *Study of the Channels and Collaterals (Jing luo xue)* 经络学. Shanghai: Shanghai Science & Technology Press, 1984.

Meng Shu-Jiang. *Study of Febrile Diseases (Wen bing xue)* 温病学. Shanghai: Shanghai Science & Technology Press, 1985.

Xi Yong-Jiang. *Study of Acupuncture and Moxibustion Technique (Zhen fa jiu fa xue)* 针法灸法学. Shanghai: Shanghai Science & Technology Press, 1985.

Yang Chang-Sen. *Acupuncture and Moxibustion Therapeutics (Zhen jiu zhi liao xue)* 针灸治疗学. Shanghai: Shanghai Science & Technology Press, 1985.

Yang Ji-Zhou. *Great Compendium of Acupuncture and Moxibustion (Zhen jiu da cheng)* 针灸大成. Beijing: Peoples Health Publishing Company, 1955. [Originally published in 1602.]

Yang Jia-San. *Study of the Acupuncture Points (Shu xue xue)* 腧穴学. Shanghai: Shanghai Science & Technology Press, 1984.

Yin Hui-He. *Basic Theory of Traditional Chinese Medicine (Zhong yi ji chu li lun)* 中医基础理论. Shanghai: Shanghai Science & Technology Press, 1984.

Zhang Bo-Yu. *Internal Medicine in Traditional Chinese Medicine (Zhong yi nei ke xue)* 中医内科学. Shanghai: Shanghai Science & Technology Press, 1985.

Zhang Zhong-Jing. *Discussion of Cold-induced Disorders (Shang han lun)* 伤寒论. Edited by Li Pei-Sheng. Beijing: People's Health Publishing Company, 1987. [Originally written in 3rd century A.D.]

Zhang Zhong-Jing. *Essentials of the Golden Cabinet with Annotations (Jin gui yao lue quan jie)* 金匮要略诠解. Edited by Liu Du-zhou. Tianjin: Tianjin Science & Technology Press, 1984. [Originally written in 3rd century A.D.]

Journals

Beijing College of Chinese Medicine. *Journal of the Beijing College of Traditional Chinese Medicine (Beijing zhong yi xue yuan xue bao)* 北京中医学院学报.

China Academy of Chinese Medicine. *Chinese Acupuncture and Moxibustion (Zhong guo zhen jiu)* 中国针灸.

China Academy of Chinese Medicine. *Journal of Traditional Chinese Medicine (Zhong yi za zhi)* 中医杂志.

Guangzhou College of Chinese Medicine. *Journal of the Guangzhou College of Traditional Chinese Medicine (Guangzhou zhong yi xue yuan xue bao)* 广州中医学院学报.

Shanghai Academy of Chinese Medicine. *Shanghai Journal of Acupuncture and Moxibustion (Shanghai zhen jiu za zhi)* 上海针灸杂志.

Shanghai College of Chinese Medicine. *Journal of the Shanghai College of Traditional Chinese Medicine (Shanghai zhong yi xue yuan xue bao)* 上海中医学院学报.

Tianjin College of Chinese Medicine. *Journal of the Tianjin College of Traditional Chinese Medicine (Tianjin zhong yi xue yuan xue bao)* 天津中医学院学报.

Point Index

General Index